Health Status Measurement
A brief but critical introduction

Crispin Jenkinson
Health Services Research Unit
University of Oxford

and

Hannah McGee
Department of Psychology
Royal College of Surgeons in Ireland

RADCLIFFE MEDICAL PRESS

Radcliffe Medical Press Ltd
18 Marcham Road, Abingdon, Oxon OX14 1AA

British Library Cataloguing in Publication Data
A catalogue record for this book is available from the British Library.

ISBN 1 85775 228 7

Typeset by Joshua Associates Ltd, Oxford
Printed and bound by Biddles Ltd, Guildford and King's Lynn

Contents

Preface

The evaluation of health and medical care increasingly incorporates patient-based assessments. This is a far cry from traditional medical evaluation which relied upon clinical assessment and the results of blood tests, X-rays and the results of other technical measures. Patient report was regarded as 'soft data' that was inaccurate and unreliable. However, whilst measuring subjective health status is not a simple undertaking, the importance of it cannot be underestimated. Any evaluation of health care interventions which ignores how patients feel can provide only a limited account of the success or otherwise of treatment.

The purpose of this book is to introduce readers to the terminology used in the arena of subjective health status measurement as well as the issues to be considered when using this form of assessment. The potential applications and benefits of health status measurement are discussed and the requirements of measures across different applications considered. The book introduces the reader to the fundamentals of psychometrics, the science of measuring mental and subjective phenomena which are used in the construction of questionnaires in this field. Some of the most widely used instruments are then critically reviewed. Finally, consideration is given as to how measures should be evaluated and chosen for inclusion in studies, and how readers might usefully evaluate published articles that include such material. It is intended that this book will provide not only an introduction to this area but also provide a critical sense of some of the issues in health status measurement. A glossary of commonly used terms is included as well as a guide to other texts which deal in greater detail with some of the subjects considered here.

Crispin Jenkinson
Hannah McGee
August 1998

Acknowledgements

We are grateful to a large number of people for their help, either direct or indirect, in the preparation of this book. Many of our colleagues and friends have given of their time and expertise and we wish to extend our grateful thanks to them all. In particular, we wish to acknowledge Ray Fitzpatrick, Andrew Garratt, Danny Ruta, Richard Layte, Nick Black, Katherine Watson, Matthew Clayton, Ralph Dennison, Andrew Williams, Ann Bowling, John Browne, Charles Duncan, David Fletcher, Paul Montgomery, Ciaran O'Boyle, Linda O'Connell, Brian, Robert and Don O'Boyle, Colin Paice, Jane Barlow, Viv Peto, Lucie Wright, Martin Vessey, Dympna Waldron and Sue Ziebland. Errors and omissions in the text are, of course, our own.

This book is dedicated to our parents

Mary and Keith Jenkinson
Mary McGee and the memory of Thomas McGee

1
Health status measurement: a guide to the text

Introduction

The ways in which medical treatments are evaluated and medicine is practised are changing. Historically, unsystematic observations of clinical practice were the basis of professional knowledge. Thus, the value of diagnostic tests and treatment was not based on rigorous or systematic evaluation.[1] Consequently, there were, and indeed still are, enormous variations in medical practice not only between countries but between different geographical areas of the same country.[2] Such uncertainty about the benefit of medical interventions remains common but the growing trend toward evidence-based medicine[3] has begun to introduce a more critical assessment of evidence. Limited resources and ever-increasing demands for health care mean that there is a growing awareness that medical treatments should be provided only when there is information available that they are effective. In order to determine whether a treatment is effective, it is necessary to systematically measure the outcome of the intervention. Traditionally, outcomes of treatment have been evaluated in terms of mortality and radiological, clinical and laboratory assessments, but there is a growing belief that, in many instances, potentially the most important outcome measure is to be gained from the patient's perspective.[4] This has led to the search for instruments, in the form of questionnaires, which can measure subjective health status in a meaningful and reliable way.

Subjective health status questionnaires can, of course, be used outside the arena of treatment regime evaluation, but their growing importance in this field has been the major impetus to their development and application. The purpose of this text is to introduce newcomers to the field of outcomes research, by outlining both the applications within clinical medicine and elsewhere to which such measures may be put and the ways in which such measures are constructed, tested and applied.

What is subjective health status?

There has been a massive increase in the use of subjective health indicators in the medical literature in the last 20 years. The increase in the number of papers including some aspect of subjective health status or so-called 'quality of life' reflects a growing interest on the part of physicians and health researchers in utilizing the patient's viewpoint in formulating treatment plans and monitoring the quality of medical care outcomes.[5] As more of the population experience the limitations of ageing, chronic illness and disability, due to increased lifespan, a need has developed for a more humanistic form of health care which incorporates a systematic assessment of the patient's perceptions.

Interest in subjective patient-based assessment is also in keeping with the World Health Organization's (WHO) definition of health: 'Health is a state of complete physical, mental and social well-being and not merely absence of disease'.[6] This definition underscores the importance of including the functional, social, cultural, subjective and sociopsychological variables that impact on role performance, independent living and perceived well-being in any elaborated conception of health. Later, a WHO scientific group added that personal 'autonomy' was also critical to quality of life.[7]

Health-related quality of life is a concept that attempts to encompass the spirit of the WHO definition of health by incorporating both personal health status and social well-being in assessing the health of individuals and populations. The concept has not been well defined because it evolved from a loosely integrated body of research on health status, functional performance and social well-being. This body of work assimilated studies of physical conditions like diagnostic category, health status and functional ability; psychological factors like pain, emotions, locus of control, sense of self-worth and intellectual functioning; social variables like social role performance and support networks; and composite measures of these elements. Although there is no agreed single definition of health-related quality of life, the definitions available generally concur on the components that ought to be included: general health, cognitive function, mental health, emotional state, subjective well-being, life satisfaction and social support. In the relatively pragmatic field of health status measurement such a general view of what constitutes health-related quality of life has tended to dominate, though not without criticism that the field tends to lack theory. More philosophical debates about the meaning and value of health are rehearsed elsewhere.[8, 9, 10]

The purpose of this book

This text introduces readers to the terminology used in this field as well as to the issues to be considered when using this form of assessment. Chapter 2 considers the potential applications and benefits of health status measurement. The number of applications is wide but the requirements of measures can differ across applications. Chapter 3 discusses the requirements of measures of health status and provides definitions for the most important standards of validation of such instruments. Chapters 4 and 5 critically review a number of established health status profiles and index measures. Those discussed are amongst the most widely used generic measures (i.e. instruments that can be used with a wide variety of patient groups), but the issues raised often need to be considered when utilizing any health status measure. Chapter 6 discusses the pros and cons of disease-specific measures and the process of developing and validating such a measure. The final chapter suggests a framework for reviewing papers in which health status measures have been used which we hope will enable students, researchers and clinicians to make informed assessments of the appropriateness of questionnaires used and the subsequent interpretation. This book provides not only an introduction to this potentially invaluable area but also provides a critical sense of some of the limitations of which the reader should be aware.

References

1   Evidence-based Working Group (1992) Evidence-based medicine: a new approach to teaching the practice of medicine. *Journal of the American Medical Association.* **268**: 2420–5.
2   Lockett T (1997) *Evidence-Based and Cost-Effective Medicine for the Uninitiated.* Radcliffe Medical Press, Oxford.
3   Sackett DL, Richardson WS, Rosenberg W, Haynes RB (1997) *Evidence Based Medicine. How to teach and practise EBM.* Churchill Livingstone, London.

4 Jenkinson C (1995) Measuring the outcomes of medical care: possibilities and limitations. *Social Science and Medicine.* **41**: 1395–401.

5 Geigle BS, Jones SB (1990) Outcomes measurement: a report from the front. *Inquiry.* **27**: 7–13.

6 World Health Organization (1984) The constitution of the World Health Organization. *WHO Chronicle.* **1**: 13.

7 World Health Organization (1984) *Uses of Epidemiology in Aging.* Technical Report Series 706. World Health Organization, Geneva.

8 Nordenfelt L (ed) (1994) *Concepts and Measurement of Quality of Life in Health Care.* Kluwer Academic, Boston.

9 Nussbaum M, Sen A (1993) *The Quality of Life.* Oxford University Press, Oxford.

10 Clayton M, Williams A (1994) Subjective health status and distributive justice. In: *Measuring Health and Medical Outcomes* (ed C Jenkinson), UCL Press, London.

2
Applications of health status measurement

Introduction

Health status assessment extends the information available to the general public, to patients, to health professionals, to health-funding agencies and to policy makers to help them evaluate the impact of illness and the treatments provided to manage it. The information obtained may be considered in great detail in circumstances such as randomized controlled trials where competing therapies with often similar clinical benefits are being compared for their positive or negative impact on a wider range of health considerations. This can influence the adoption or otherwise of new methods of treating disease. At the other extreme, health status information about particular diseases or treatments reaches the general public, after it has been interpreted, through the popular press or information provided by medical charities or other health care agencies. This provides, to the community at large, a better under-standing of the impacts of various diseases upon quality of life and daily activities as well as giving some sense of the efficacy of available treatments.

Health status measures are completed by individuals themselves, rather than by health professionals on their behalf. Such assessment attempts to move the focus of outcomes evaluation from technical measures of success assessed by health professionals to those outcomes valued by patients. This chapter outlines the main purposes for which health status assessment can be used. These are concerned with the health care delivery system – randomized controlled trials and individual patient care, and with the wider context – population studies and resource allocation decision making

Randomized controlled trials

The randomized controlled trial (RCT) is a longitudinal study in which participants are allocated to 'study' and 'control' groups. In its simplest form, patients in the study group receive active treatment and those in the control group do not (the latter group instead receiving a placebo, i.e. sham or inert treatment). Alternatively, those in the study group receive a newly developed treatment whilst those in the control group receive an established treatment. Patients are randomly allocated between the groups (in terms of age, sex, social class, etc.) to minimize bias. Interventions evaluated using this methodology range from new medications and surgical interventions to new methods of service delivery such as, for example, the provision of health care in the home rather than in hospital.[1] Health status assessment is increasingly used in RCTs where outcomes other than survival are of interest.[2] This seems long overdue given that many currently used therapies have no effect on life expectancy but are designed to improve patient health status; for instance, joint replacement surgery aims to reduce pain and restore the individual's ability to perform a range of activities of daily living.

Health status measures are also used in trials where the primary outcome of interest is a clinical variable. Thus, they are often included as secondary measures; clinical outcomes such as reduced tumour size or increased cardiac capacity are considered the primary indicators of success, with health status differences providing insight into the potential effects the competing treatments may have on quality of life. Furthermore, in situations where clinical outcomes are equivalent quality of life data can be used to select between competing therapies. Guidelines for reporting results of health status assessments in clinical trials have been developed.[3]

Many trials are international and, consequently, questionnaires must be available in numerous languages. Great care must be taken in translating such measures to ensure that the meaning of the questions is not lost. Obviously, if the questionnaires used in different countries are not equivalent then the data cannot be aggregated. Issues in the cross-cultural adaptation of measures must be considered when selecting a measure for an international trial. These important issues are considered in detail elsewhere.[4]

Individual patient care

Health status assessment can be used to improve individual care in a number of ways. First, health status assessment may be useful as a means of providing a unique patient perspective on disease and its impact. A large body of evidence demonstrates that health professionals are poor judges of how aspects of life quality are affected by illness and treatment for individual patients. Typically, professionals are poorer judges of the less observable aspects of health status such as psychological functioning. While they may underestimate the level of distress or concern associated with a patient's condition, they are also less able to perceive positive aspects of health status than are patients.[5] Health status measurement may usefully complement clinical evaluation by health professionals since it provides a broader picture of patient functioning. In fact, the process of collecting such data may in itself improve professional–patient communication. The Dartmouth COOP charts have been designed to provide a brief overview of health status suited to completion as part of a general practitioner consultation.[6] Both patients and physicians have reported that using the charts results in improved interaction and treatment.[7]

A second use of health status assessment is in screening patients to evaluate their needs for particular services. This type of approach has been used most frequently in screening for psychological distress. For instance, cardiac patients have been screened for anxiety and depression and patients scoring above pre-determined cut-off points referred for specialist cardiac rehabilitation services.[8] The two major challenges to the use of health status instruments in this way relate to measurement properties of the instrument and to the use to which such information will be put. To be useful, screening instruments must be accurate, i.e. they must be able to identify both those individuals who exhibit the phenomenon in question (test sensitivity) and those who do not exhibit the phenomenon (test specificity). The level of development of health status measures at present is such that there is little available evidence on sensitivity and specificity. We are not in a position to determine what values for concepts such as energy, social support or daily activities constitute legitimate cut-off points, levels below which intervention is needed to improve function in these areas.

Related to this is the second challenge. The use of health status instruments to screen individuals should be accompanied by a plan to provide appropriate interventions for those identified as having difficulty in an investigated dimension. For the areas just listed, it may be difficult to decide what form of intervention should be provided to achieve one's aim or, indeed, it may be that the expense involved in providing a specific intervention prohibits its availability. Another means of justifying screening using health status measures would be to demonstrate that information provided on patient status to clinicians improved the clinical management or outcome of the patient. However, there is little evidence to show that this actually does happen. For example, in a randomized study of rheumatoid arthritis,[9] patients completed health status measures either at the beginning and end of a one-year study (control group) or four times over the year. The latter group was divided into those whose results were sent quarterly to their treating physicians (experimental group) or those whose physicians did not receive the information (attention placebo). There were no changes in a range of process or outcome parameters across groups at the end of the year, i.e. medication changes, referral to other services, patient satisfaction or health status.

Finally, when patients present with health problems there is increasingly a range of possible options rather than one 'best practice'. These options often have differing benefits and drawbacks. Evaluation of patient health status and preferences may guide the professional and patient to selecting the option which is most suited to the individual. For example, benign prostatic hyperplasia, a condition of bladder irritation and obstruction affecting many older men, can be treated surgically or medically. Surgery may resolve symptoms but also involves some risk of permanent sexual or urinary dysfunction or perioperative death. Medical management may involve lesser resolution of symptoms and also some unpleasant side-effects of medications such as in the case of hormonal treatments. It seems likely that, in this instance, those with relatively minor symptoms or the very frail elderly are more likely to adopt medical management rather than surgery. Health status assessment may provide systematic information on the health status of patients which can aid this decision making. However, to date, such faith has rarely been put in such measurement.

Population studies

The health status of whole populations or populations defined by particular characteristics, e.g. patients following myocardial infarction, can be assessed. General population assessment provides information on the health profile and possible health care needs of the community at large. Health status can be considered as it relates to salient issues for the population such as gender, age, socioeconomic status, ethnicity and place of residence. It has been suggested that such information can be used to determine what services are needed, where they are needed and to whom they should be targeted. While some argue that this information has the potential to be very useful for health planning, it would seem likely that much more detailed data than those provided by health status measures would need to be collected as variations in health status do not give any clear indication of the needs of the population being studied. Such data may tell us that a given area or group has worse health but does not tell us why.

Population studies can be used to gain normative data for a measure. In the UK a number of large regional samples have been assessed using the SF-36 Questionnaire in postal surveys.[10,11] Information from such population studies provides comparison data from which to judge the difficulties associated with particular diseases or treatments. For example, comparison of women referred for breast reduction surgery with population norms on the SF-36 health status questionnaire demonstrated that they experienced significant levels of pain which was resolved by surgery.[12]

Resource allocation

Since the demand for and cost of health care continue to rise, there is an increasing need for an explicit and rational method of resource allocation in systems which cannot afford to fund every health intervention. A major driving force in the development of health status instruments has been the search for ways to inform and justify rationing decisions. The rationale is that treatments can be evaluated with regard to the impact they have on health status. This information is combined with analysis of the cost of different treatments in order to identify the best value for money when funding health services. The most widely used health status assessment concept in resource allocation considerations is the quality-adjusted life-year (QALY), described in detail in Chapter 5. In some situations, the comparison for resource allocation purposes is of alternative treatments for the same individual. In other situations, the comparison is across treatments for a range of different health problems.

There has been much discussion of the moral and ethical acceptability of utilitarian approaches to health resource allocation such as QALYs. On one side, there is the view that since decisions about scarce health resources have to be and are being made, these measures provide some explicit method of obtaining the best value for money. The counterargument is that of equity – that individuals are entitled to equal access to treatment and that it should not be determined by the particular health problem one experiences. Some attempts have been made to use health status instruments to make explicit priorities for funding. In the USA, the state of Oregon attempted to generate and prioritize a list of services it would fund on behalf of its citizens in the 1980s. Using wide-ranging community consultation and debate and including a health status questionnaire (the General Well-being Scale) to assist planning, they prioritized from a list of 1680 health care procedures they would fund at state level. In doing this, they also by definition made explicit those procedures that were uneconomic to fund. These included some services for babies born prematurely and also organ replacement procedures. However, there was a very negative community response to the completed priority listing, despite its development with community participation. The list was initially reorganized to take account of the public response but then in 1992 the Oregon Health Services Commission eliminated any consideration of quality of life.[13]

Attempting to make rationing decisions based on quality of life may seem unpleasant or difficult, but removing it altogether seems almost absurd. Of course, rationing goes on whether there is community involvement or not. Some are, of course, happy to see rationing, or so-called 'priority setting', undertaken without recourse to community values or the application of scientific principles. Writing in the *British Medical Journal* in 1991, Sir Raymond Hoffenberg remarked 'If services are to be limited I would rather see it done implicitly – unstated, unwritten, unacknowledged – in the curious and not inhumane way in which such matters are managed in the United Kingdom'.[14] Such a view is increasingly seen as being out of step by those health care managers holding budgets that are insufficient to buy all the services they would wish to provide.

Summary

Health status assessments can be used for a variety of purposes ranging from informing individual health care to guiding resource allocation in the health system. The selection of measures to use will be influenced by the purpose of the study. The requirements and the types of measures available for these different applications are discussed in the following chapters.

References

1 Shepperd S, Doll H, Jenkinson C (1997) Randomised controlled trials. In: *Assessment and Evaluation of Health and Medical Care* (ed C Jenkinson), Open University Press, Buckingham.

2 Staquet MJ, Hays RD, Fayers PM (eds) (1998) *Quality of Life Assessment in Clinical Trials. Methods and practice.* Oxford University Press, Oxford.

3 Staquet MJ, Berzon RJ, Osoba D, Machin D (1998) Guidelines for reporting results of quality of life assessments in clinical trials. In: *Quality of Life Assessment in Clinical Trials. Methods and practice* (eds MJ Staquet, RD Hays, PM Fayers), Oxford University Press, Oxford.

4 Bullinger M (1995) International validation and testing of quality of life scales in relation to Germany. In: *Quality of Life and Health: concepts, methods and applications* (eds I Guggenmoos-Holzman, K Bloomfield, H Brener, U Flick), Blackwell Wissenschaft, Berlin.

5 Sprangers MA, Aaronson NK (1992) The role of health care providers and significant others in evaluating the quality of life of patients with chronic disease: a review. *Journal of Clinical Epidemiology.* **45**: 743–60.

6 Wasson JH, Keller A, Rubenstein L, Hays R, Nelson E, Johnson D and the Dartmouth Primary Care COOP Project (1992) Benefits and obstacles of health status assessments in ambulatory settings: the clinician's point of view. *Medical Care.* **30** (suppl): MS42–MS49.

7 Kraus N (1991) *The InterStudy Quality Edge, Volume 1, No. 1.* InterStudy, Excelsior, Minneapolis.

8 Oldridge N, Guyatt G, Jones N, Crowne J, Singer J (1991) Effects on quality of life with comprehensive rehabilitation after acute myocardial infarction. *American Journal of Cardiology.* **67**: 1084–9.

9 Kazis LE, Anderson JJ, Meenan RF (1988) Health status information in clinical practice: the development and testing of patient profile reports. *Journal of Rheumatology.* **15**: 338–44.

10 Jenkinson C, Coulter A, Wright L (1993) Short form 36 (SF-36) health survey questionnaire: normative data for adults of working age. *British Medical Journal.* **306**: 1437–40.

11 Brazier JE, Harper R, Jones NMB, *et al.* (1992) Validating the SF-36 health survey questionnaire: a new outcome measure for primary care. *British Medical Journal.* **305**: 160–4.

12 Klassen A, Fitzpatrick R, Jenkinson C, Goodacre T (1996) Should breast reduction be rationed? A comparison of the health status of patients before and after surgery. *British Medical Journal.* **313**: 454–6.

13 Kaplan RM (1994) Value judgement in the Oregon Medicaid Experiment. *Medical Care*. **10**: 975–88.
14 Editorial (1991) Rationing: the search for sunlight. *British Medical Journal*. **303**: 1561–2.

3
Requirements of measures

Introduction

Measuring subjective health state is a relatively recent phenomenon. Historically, medicine relied on traditional clinical, radiological and laboratory tests. Patient report was not systematically collected and analysed. The relatively slow growth in interest in measuring subjective health outcomes was in part due to the view of some medical researchers and clinicians that measuring subjective experience was either very difficult or impossible and that such an undertaking could never really be based upon scientific principles and procedures. Consequently, traditional medical assessments gained the status of 'hard data' and patient-based material as 'soft data' – the latter, rather pejorative term, implying the data were, one assumes, either redundant or simply inaccurate. Needless to say, anyone who has ever tried to develop a questionnaire will have found the process less straightforward than might initially be imagined. Furthermore, those who have attempted to complete questionnaires which don't make sense or are repetitive or irrelevant will be aware that the superficially simple task of asking questions is an activity that is often done very badly. This is because some investigators have rather naively assumed that designing a health assessment measure or, indeed, any questionnaire requires little more than a pen, paper and common sense. However, all good-quality measurement has standards for validating and checking the results it produces and questionnaire design is no different.

A number of issues must be considered when designing a questionnaire or assessing any given instrument for inclusion in a study. The purpose of this chapter is not to provide a definitive guide to questionnaire design but to introduce readers to some of the more essential aspects of questionnaire validation and assessment, as well as the terminology used in this area. For those who wish to go further, some excellent texts have been produced to guide people through the development, validation and psychometrics of this area.[1,2] However, these texts do assume some knowledge of the field, which is covered below.

Measurement theory: nominal, ordinal, interval and ratio scales

Most health assessment questionnaires are based upon scales. A scale is a graded system of categories, of which there are broadly four types which have very different characteristics.

Nominal scales distinguish classes of objects. For example, the classification of sex into 1 = male and 2 = female is a nominal scale. A more complex nominal scale is the International Classification of Diseases, where numerical values classify all diagnoses and presenting problems. There is no hierarchy implied by the values ascribed, so in the example of sex the codes 1 = female and 2 = male could be as meaningfully used as 1 = male and 2 = female. Statistical analysis of such data must be restricted to simple cross-tabulations and frequencies.

Ordinal scales are scales on which classes or objects are ordered on a continuum (for example, from Best to Worst). No indication is given as to the distance between values, although a hierarchy is assumed to exist. Thus, when classifying an illness into 1 = mild, 2 = moderate and 3 = severe, it cannot be assumed that the extent of difference between mild and moderate is similar to the difference between moderate and severe. Rank order correlation is an appropriate statistical analysis for such data. Tabular representation of data is appropriate but even simple descriptive statistics (such as means and standard deviations) based on such data should ideally be avoided as results can be misleading. For example, if the real 'difference' between 1 and 2 is greater than that between 2 and 3, calculating a mean on the scores 1, 2 and 3 will not be sensitive to this fact. However, whilst the purists may promote such principles most researchers adopt a more pragmatic approach and consequently break these rules. Indeed, it has been argued that the errors produced by such analyses are generally small.[3] A large number of health status measures in use today adopt ordinal scales on which numerous (sometimes quite inappropriate) statistics are applied! However, scaling procedures are often used (see reference 2 for information on psychometric scaling procedures) in order to improve the numerical characteristics of response scales and attempts are made to convert what are effectively ordinal response categories into interval level response scales. Such scaling procedures are discussed elsewhere and are beyond the scope of this text.[4]

Interval scales are designed on the assumption that the scale is ordered and the distances between values on one part of the scale are equal in distance to the distances between values on another part of the scale. Temperature is measured on such a scale. However, interval scales lack an absolute baseline anchorpoint. For example, a thermometer is an interval scale but it is not possible to assume that 60°F is twice as hot as 30°F (because 0°F is not as cold as it can get). Subtraction and addition of such data are appropriate, but ideally not division or multiplication. Pearson correlation, factor analysis and discriminant analysis are appropriate analysis techniques. In health status measurement, it is not uncommon to see researchers converting ordinal responses to interval scales. Thus, attempts are made to weight responses rather than simply to use arbitrary codes, such as 0 = no health problems, 1 = some health problems and 2 = many health problems. However, there is a considerable body of evidence that weighting schemes do not generally improve the accuracy and reliability of most health status measures and they often seem to provide little more than a pseudoscientific level of accuracy that is unrealistic in this area of measurement.

Ratio scales are similar to interval scales but with an absolute zero point, so that ratios between values can be meaningfully defined. Thus, time, weight and height are all examples of ratio scales. For example, it is perfectly acceptable to assume that 48 hours is twice as long a time period as 24 hours. All forms of statistical analysis may be used with such data, although care should be taken in the choice of methods, depending on the spread of the data. Ideally, data should be normally distributed (i.e. follow the 'bell' curve) if parametric statistics (i.e. statistical tests which assume normality in the distribution of data) are to be used, although in practice this rule is frequently broken. However, such rule breaking can mean results are less than robust. It is something of a moot point as to whether any health status measure could truly claim to be a ratio scale, although the weighting schemes used for health economic measures may be regarded as falling into this category (see Chapter 5). However, in reality, we can never be certain if the zero points are truly accurate.

Ideally measures should be developed using interval or ratio scales, but this is no easy task in the social sciences. Measures of health status can never truly be regarded as fulfilling the requirements of these forms of measurement.[4] Consequently, attempts are made to ensure that the results of measures at least fulfil certain criteria. It is to these important criteria that we now turn our attention.

Validity and reliability

Validity

A valid assessment is one that measures what it claims to measure. The evaluation of the validity of a measure usually involves comparison with some standardized criterion or criteria. This is no easy thing in the social sciences as there are rarely 'gold standards' against which measures can be compared. However, a number of standard criteria for validity are usually assessed for any properly constructed questionnaire. Essentially, there are four aspects to validity: face validity, content validity, criterion validity and construct validity.

Face validity refers to whether items on a questionnaire appear both appropriate to the phenomenon being measured and to make sense, as well as being easily understood. This may seem a simple enough test for a questionnaire to pass, but there are ambiguities in some of the most respected and well-utilized measures. For example, in the next chapter some problems with the wording of the Sickness Impact Profile and the SF-36, two of the most utilized measures of health status, will be discussed.

Content validity refers to choice of, and relative importance given to, items on a questionnaire. In a matter as fundamental as the selection of items, a number of approaches are available to the potential designer. Broadly speaking, items can be developed by the researcher, from searches of the literature, from studies of lay people, patient surveys or any combination of these. Whichever is used, it is important that items appropriate to the phenomenon under investigation are chosen and if they are weighted in some way, that the weights reflect the perceived level of difficulty or health problem. Thus, if one were to interview several hundred people and ask them to nominate the things that contribute to their well-being a vast array of statements would be selected. Only a limited number could be used in any questionnaire and one must try to ensure that the items chosen will be appropriate to a large number of people. Thus, good health would seem to be an important aspect of well-being and one could easily imagine statements on this being included in a health or quality of life questionnaire. However, how healthy one's pet piglet may or may not be would not be an appropriate item as it would apply to so few people; neither would a question on how enjoyable breakfast was last Sunday as, for most people, most of the time, this will not indicate to any great extent level of health or quality of life. Similarly, if the items are weighted one would expect there to be a predictable hierarchy to some weightings, such as a greater weight for 'I am depressed all the time' than for 'I feel a little bit miserable on occasion'. Assessment of content validity is not a technical undertaking, but rather the application of common sense to the questionnaire under consideration. Some established questionnaires do not fully pass this test; for example, weights in the Nottingham Health Profile can lead to some counterintuitive results (with people with a variety of minor difficulties in mobility gaining similar scores to those who are unable to walk) whilst the Sickness Impact Profile, which is a measure of the impact of disease upon perceived health, does not contain a dimension to measure pain, which is surely one of the most salient aspects of a large number of illnesses. These issues are explored in greater depth in Chapter 4.

Construct validity is an important aspect of validity, especially in the social sciences where the variable being measured cannot be observed directly. It refers to where hypotheses are generated and a questionnaire is tested to determine if it actually reflects these prior hypotheses. For example, the construct validity of the SF-36 has been checked to ensure that certain groups (e.g. older, lower social classes, those with illnesses) would gain lower (i.e. worse) scores than other groups (e.g. younger, higher social classes, those without illnesses). Construct validity is sometimes divided into convergent validity and discriminant validity. For convergent validity one would expect results from a measure to be related to other variables and measures of the same construct. Discriminant validity is the mirror image of convergent validity in that it is assumed that results will not be related when the questionnaire data are compared to other data measuring distinct and unrelated concepts.

Criterion validity refers to the ability of an instrument to correspond with other measures held up as 'gold standards'. In practice, few studies can truly claim to have evaluated criterion validity as 'gold standards' are hard to find in this area of research. Results from questionnaires have been compared with clinical criteria; for example, results from the Arthritis Impact Measurement Scales (AIMS)[5,6] were compared with various rheumatological measures and results from the Parkinson's Disease Questionnaire compared to various clinical assessments of the disease progression as well as to results on another health status measure.[7] However, given that subjective health questionnaires are designed to measure different aspects of health than those tapped by traditional measures, such assessments can really only give a very general impression that measures are related. It would be worrying if clinical assessments and subjective health status measures were completely contradictory, but likewise it would be surprising if they correlated perfectly.

Questionnaire results on one measure are often compared with those of another. Usually little more is sought than a set of generally predicted associations, but from time to time one measure is expected to closely reflect the results of another. Usually this is when a shorter form of a measure is being compared to the original. For example, the results of the physical and mental health summary scales from the 36-item SF-36 have been compared with results from the 12-item version of the questionnaire and have been found to be almost identical.[8] The 'gold standard' in this instance is the longer form measure and perhaps, in the field of health status measurement, it is only when comparing longer and shorter forms that proclaim to measure identical phenomena that one could really ever say that one measure truly was a 'gold standard'. This form of criterion validity is sometimes referred to as concurrent validity (comparing results from two measures administered at the same time). Another, though relatively rarely used form of criterion validity is predictive validity where results on one measure are expected to be predictive of some future event or outcome. Kazis and colleagues used the Arthritis Impact Measurement Scales and examined the relationship between health and mortality in a five-year study of patients with rheumatoid arthritis.[9] They found that subjective health reports were predictive of death with a significant linear trend for death and scores on both the general health and physical functioning dimensions of the questionnaire.

Reliability

One would hope that a measure that fulfils the requirements for validity would also be reliable. Questionnaires must be reliable over time. Thus, they should produce the same, or very similar results, on two or more administrations to the same respondents, provided, of course, there is good reason to believe that the health status of the patients has not changed. As with validity, there are a number of methods of assessing reliability. The most commonly used method is referred to as internal reliability or internal consistency reliability and is measured using the Cronbach's alpha statistic[10] (for items with more than two response categories, such as 'Never', 'Sometimes', 'Always') and the Kuder-

Richardson (KR-20) test (for items with two response categories, such as 'Yes' or 'No'). In practice, the alpha statistic, which was derived from the KR-20 test, is used for both types of response categories and produces very similar results on dichotomous data, as does the KR-20 formula. Internal consistency involves testing for homogeneity, which assumes that there are correlations between items in a scale which are not the product of random chance but reflect a real patterning as to how the questions are answered. Alpha statistics below 0.5 are regarded as low and would suggest that items in a scale are not all tapping the same underlying area of interest. Alpha statistics above 0.9 have been taken to mean that a measure has very high internal reliability and can be used at the level of individual analysis (rather than only at the level of group analysis). However, some would suggest that such high alpha values would indicate that effectively the same question is being asked more than once. Another potential criticism of internal reliability testing is that good results do not necessarily mean that a measure is reliable over time. It does seem a little unlikely that a measure would be internally reliable yet produce unreliable results on separate occasions, although there is the possibility of a systematic shift of responses (due, perhaps, to familiarity and greater understanding of the questionnaire) which could lead to this situation. Consequently, researchers assess not only internal reliability but also test-retest reliability.

In test-retest reliability the questionnaire is administered on two occasions separated by a few days. Ideally respondents should not have changed in any way between the two administrations of the questionnaire and consequently the two administrations should produce almost identical results. The difficulty with such a method of validating a questionnaire is that it is often uncertain whether results that may indicate a questionnaire is unreliable are in fact no more than a product of real change in health status or whether the respondent's familiarity with the questionnaire may lead to changes in their responses.

Sensitivity to change

It is essential that evaluative instruments are able to detect change and the level of this change is interpretable in some way. The sensitivity to change or 'responsiveness' of an instrument is a very important criterion to consider when selecting measures. However, it has not, until relatively recently, received a great amount of attention. In part this is because researchers could present before and after treatment data and calculate whether any change was statistically significant (i.e. not a product of chance variation). Whilst this was traditionally commonplace it is unsatisfactory. It is possible to find a statistically significant difference in scores on a questionnaire before and after treatment, but it need not be at all clear that the difference means very much to either clinicians or patients. Consequently, more sophisticated ways of assessing change have been developed.

The effect size statistic is the most commonly cited interpretation of change scores.[11] This is usually calculated by subtracting the mean before treatment with that gained after treatment and dividing the result with the baseline standard deviation. This can be expressed mathematically as:

$$ES = \frac{m_1 - m_2}{SD_1}$$

where m_1 is the pre-treatment mean, m_2 the post and SD_1 is the pre-treatment standard deviation. The before treatment scores are effectively used as a proxy for control group scores. This approach treats the effect size as a standard measure of change in a 'before and after' study context. Note that as the purpose of the statistic is to give some idea of the magnitude of the change rather than the statistical significance the standard deviation at baseline is used rather than the standard deviation of the differences between means.[12] An effect size of 1.00 is equivalent to a change of one standard deviation in the sample. As a benchmark for assessing change, it has been suggested that an effect size of 0.2 is small, 0.5 is moderate and 0.8 is large.[13] However, whilst these cut-off points are useful as a general rule some caution is needed in interpretation. For example, it is possible for a very sensitive instrument to indicate large effect sizes for what are subjectively relatively modest changes.

The manner of calculating the effect size as documented above has been criticized. Two other widely used approaches are documented here. Liang et al.[14] have suggested a modification to the calculation of the effect size, which they refer too as the standardized response mean (SRM) statistic. They argue that the baseline standard deviation does not incorporate response variance (i.e. variations between respondents as to responses at baseline and then at follow-up) and therefore it does not contain information on the ability of the instrument to detect change over time. Consequently, they suggest using the same numerator as that used in the effect size but the standard deviation of the mean change score as the denominator. This SRM has been advocated as superior to the effect size as calculated above in the assessment of the sensitivity to change when comparing various instruments because it takes account of response variance that is likely to vary between instruments. In practice, the differences in results between the two methods are often fairly small.

A variant on the SRM has been suggested by Guyatt and colleagues.[15] They suggest that sensitivity to change is in part a function of the variability in score changes for stable subjects. In other words a measure has an ability to pick up real changes but also is likely to pick up 'noise'. They suggest the 'responsiveness index' which is calculated by dividing the mean change of those patients who report improvement regarded as clinically important by the variability of patients reporting no change. The stable subject variability is estimated by the square root of twice the mean square error. Whilst this method does account for non-specific changes or noise, it does require the researcher to specify the minimum clinically meaningful change and, consequently, has been relatively little used in the literature and the effect size and SRM are more commonly reported.

One potential problem with all the methods of assessing change outlined above is that they are primarily statistical. Other attempts have been suggested to make changes interpretable. Juniper and colleagues[16] have carried out studies trying to determine what patients believe is the minimally important change on questionnaires. Thus, people complete measures and, when change is reported, they are asked to indicate whether the level of change was unimportant, minimally important or of greater importance. From these data, it is possible to calculate the amount of change typically seen as minimally important to patients. However, one criticism of this approach is that all one need ask is whether changes are minimally important or not. This method of 'calibrating' questionnaires has not been used extensively, although it may prove an invaluable approach in the coming years as there are increasing demands to make the results of disease-specific measures more interpretable.

Content-based interpretation lends itself to both disease-specific and generic measures, whereby scores on the questionnaire are interpreted by recourse to the contents of questions. In other words, in order to gain insight into the meanings of scores one simply looks to the items and response categories to see what needs to be affirmed (or not) to lead to certain scores. Table 3.1 gives some indication of what given scores may mean in relation to the way questions have been completed on the SF-36. More detailed tables than the example shown here can, of course, be developed for all questionnaires. However, it is often possible to gain the same score by affirming very different questions. Consequently, content-based interpretation in this simple manner is not possible

A more sophisticated form of content analysis has been proposed by

Dimension (no. of items)	Low scores	High scores
Physical functioning[11]	Limited a lot in performing activities including bathing and dressing	Performs all types of physical activities without limitations due to health
Role limitations due to physical problems[4]	Problems with work or other daily activities as a result of physical health	No problems with work or other daily activities due to physical health
Role limitations due to emotional problems[3]	Problems with work or other daily activities as a result of emotional problems	No problems with work or other daily activities as a result of emotional problems
Social functioning[2]	Extreme and frequent interference with normal social activities due to physical or emotional problems	Performs normal social activities without interference due to physical or emotional problems
Mental health[5]	Feelings of nervousness and depression all the time	Feels peaceful, happy and calm all the time
Energy/vitality[4]	Feels tired and worn down all the time	Feels full of energy all the time
Bodily pain[2]	Severe and limiting bodily pain	No pain or limitations due to pain
General health perceptions[5]	Believes personal health is poor and likely to get worse	Believes personal health is excellent

Table 3.1 A guide to the interpretation of very high or very low scores on the SF-36 (adapted from Ware and Sherbourne[18]).

Ware,[17] which involves three steps. First, an item with good face validity should be chosen from a scale. Thus, the question should be easy to interpret and answers to it should give some indication of the severity of respondents' health state. Second, items on the scale should be dichotomized in a meaningful way (e.g. those who claim that they can always walk half a mile without problems and those who claim they cannot). Third, the percentage endorsing the item can be plotted against various scores on the dimension from which the item comes. An example of interpreting scores in this way is provided by Ware. Using an American population survey, he compares scores on the 'physical functioning' scale from an established questionnaire (the SF-36; *see* Chapter 4) with responses to a question asking if respondents can walk a block or more. He finds that, for example, an improvement from 45 to 55 would suggest an increase of approximately 18% of people able to walk one block. The problem with this method of interpreting data is that it places a great deal of weight upon a single question. Given that scales are developed because single questions are often viewed as unreliable measures, this can seem a rather odd way of calibrating a scale.

Questionnaires that are scaled using Guttman scaling or Rasch analysis (the latter being a form of so-called 'item response theory' or 'latent trait theory') assume linearity in what is being measured. Thus, an answer to one question infers certain predictable responses to others as there is a clear hierarchy. However, measures developed using these techniques have been used relatively infrequently because of the rather strong assumptions and difficulties in creating such scales. Interested readers can find excellent introductions to these techniques elsewhere.[4]

A method of interpretation that can be adopted with generic measures is to compare results before and after treatment with norms for the general population. For example, in one study[19] it was found that approximately 75% of sleep apnoea patients scored results on an emotional health outcome scale (the SF-36 Mental Health Component Summary[20,21]) that would have placed them in the bottom 30% of the general population. After treatment (with continuous positive airways pressure therapy), 50% of patients' scores would have placed them in the top 50% of the population. This method of interpreting data gives some insight into the meaning of scores, but does require normative data to be available and hence seems to rule out the possibility of results on disease-specific measures being calculated in this way (by definition, one cannot get normative 'population-based' data for people with a specific disease).

Summary

Subjective health measurement questionnaires are not designed to be used as substitutes for traditional measures of clinical endpoints but are intended to complement existing measures and to provide a fuller picture of health state than can be gained by clinical measures alone. However, to be useful such measures must be carefully chosen. Health status measures can provide a useful adjunct to the data traditionally obtained from mortality and morbidity statistics or from traditional clinical and laboratory assessments, but careful consideration must be given to the choice of measures. Data on the reliability and validity of measures must be assessed, as must the sensitivity to change of measures in particular patient groups. At the present state of development, more research is still required to determine the appropriateness of measures for various clinical groups and the sensitivity to change and validity of measures across community and patient samples.

References

1 Oppenheim AN (1992) *Questionnaire Design, Interviewing and Attitude Measurement.* Pinter, London.

2 Streiner D, Norman G (1995) *Health Measurement Scales: a practical guide to their development and use,* 2nd edn. Oxford University Press, Oxford.

3 Nunnally J, Bernstein I (1994) *Psychometric Theory,* 3rd edn. McGraw-Hill, New York.

4 Bowling A (1997) *Measuring Health: a review of quality of life measurement scales,* 2nd edn. Open University Press, Buckingham.

5 Meenan RF, Gertman PM, Mason JH (1980) Measuring health status in arthritis: the arthritis impact measurement scales. *Arthritis and Rheumatism.* **23**: 146–52.

6 Meenan RF, Mason JH, Anderson JJ, Guccione A, Kazis L (1992) AIMS2: The content and properties of a revised and expanded arthritis impacts measurement scales health status questionnaire. *Arthritis and Rheumatism.* **35**: 1–10.

7 Jenkinson C, Peto V, Fitzpatrick R, Greenhall R, Hyman, N (1995) Self reported functioning and well being in patients with Parkinson's disease: comparison of the Short Form Health Survey (SF-36) and the Parkinson's Disease Questionnaire (PDQ-39). *Age and Ageing.* **24**: 505–9.

8 Jenkinson C, Layte R, Jenkinson D, *et al.* (1997) A shorter form health survey: can the SF12 replicate results from the SF36 in longitudinal studies? *Journal of Public Health Medicine.* **19**: 179–86.

9 Kazis L, Anderson J, Meenan RF (1990) Health status as a predictor of mortality in rheumatoid arthritis. *Journal of Rheumatology.* **17**: 609–13.

10 Cronbach LJ (1951) Coefficient alpha and the internal structure of tests. *Psychometrika.* **16**: 297–334.

11 Lydick E, Epstein RS (1993) Interpretation of quality of life changes. *Quality of Life Research.* **2**: 221–6.

12 Kazis L , Anderson JJ, Meenan RF (1989) Effect sizes for interpreting changes in health status. *Medical Care.* **27** (suppl): S178–S189.

13 Cohen J (1977) *Statistical Power for the Behavioral Sciences.* Academic Press, New York.

14 Liang M, Fossel AH, Larson MG (1990) Comparison of five health status instruments for orthopaedic evaluation. *Medical Care.* **28**: 632–42.

15 Guyatt G, Walter S, Norman TG (1987) Measuring change over time:

assessing the usefulness of evaluative instruments. *Journal of Chronic Diseases*. **40**: 171–8.

16 Juniper E, Guyatt G, Willan A, Griffith L (1994) Determining a minimally important change in a disease specific questionnaire. *Journal of Clinical Epidemiology*. **47**: 81–7.

17 Ware J, Snow K, Kosinski M, Gandek B (1993) *SF-36 Health Survey Manual and Interpretation Guide*. The Health Institute, New England Medical Center, Boston.

18 Ware J, Sherbourne C (1992) The MOS 36–item Short Form Health Survey 1. Conceptual framework and item selection. *Medical Care*. **30**: 473–83.

19 Jenkinson C (1998) The SF-36 Physical and Mental Health Summary Scores: a guide to interpretation. *Journal of Health Services Research and Policy*. **3**: 92–6.

20 Ware JE, Kosinski M, Keller SD (1994) *SF-36 Physical and Mental Health Summary Scales: a user manual*. The Health Institute, New England Medical Center, Boston.

21 Jenkinson C, Layte R, Wright L, Coulter A (1996) *The UK SF-36: an analysis and interpretation manual*. Health Services Research Unit, Oxford.

4
Generic health status profiles

Introduction

This chapter outlines some of the most widely used generic profile measures of health status. The intention is to give potential users some idea of the characteristics and differences between regularly used profile measures. It is not intended to be an exhaustive overview of the measures available as there are so many in use. Those seeking more complete coverage should consult reference books of health status measures.[1,2,3,4] What is intended here is to provide some idea of the differences between measures which, in many respects, purport to measure similar phenomena, namely aspects of self-perceived health status.

Broadly speaking, measures of health status can be generic (i.e. they can be used across a wide range of illness conditions, as well as in healthy populations) or disease specific (designed for use with a specific patient group). Furthermore, measures can provide 'single-index measures' or a profile of health status scores, measuring areas such as emotional well-being, social functioning, pain, physical functioning, etc. In this chapter measures which provide a profile of scores and which can be used across a wide range of health states are outlined and discussed: index measures and disease-specific measures are discussed in Chapters 5 and 6.

Profile measures are preferred by those researchers who claim that health status is not a unidimensional phenomenon which can be meaningfully expressed as a single figure, but instead is composed of a variety of aspects of functioning and well-being. Health measures should ideally tap a number of areas of importance to the individuals completing them and, consequently, generic measures are designed to measure aspects which may be seen as of universal importance.

The search for comprehensive and meaningful indicators of health status has led to relatively few instruments which have had appropriate levels of reliability and validity and are also easy to administer. Whilst many instruments have been developed for specific illnesses or tap a specific aspect of ill health (such as pain or depression), the search for comprehensive measures of quality of life has been relatively unsuccessful. Ideally such a measure would be able to accurately detect differences between illness groups and be sensitive to changes over time. The most frequently reported generic health measures have been the Sickness Impact Profile,[5] the UK version of which is called the Functional Limitations Profile,[6] the Nottingham Health Profile[7, 8] and, more recently, the Dartmouth COOP Charts[9, 10] and the SF-36[11] and related 'short-form' measures such as the SF-20 and SF-12.[12]

A review of some established health profiles

The Functional Limitations Profile (FLP)

The FLP was developed from an American instrument, the Sickness Impact Profile (SIP), designed in the 1970s by Marilyn Bergner and her colleagues in Seattle. Work on the questionnaire began in 1972 and the first version appeared in 1976. A revised version of the questionnaire was published in 1981[5] and since then the questionnaire has become one of the most widely used and best known generic subjective health status questionnaires.

The SIP was developed using standard psychometric procedures. The items on the SIP were gained from a wide variety of health professionals, healthy and ill people and reviews of the existing literature. This initially led to a pool of 312 items in 14 categories. Extensive research led to this number being reduced to 136 items in 12 categories. Twenty-five judges, both health professionals and lay people, rated each item on a 15-point scale and from this exercise, weights were then devised for each item in each category. These weights reflect the relative severity of each item in a given category. Respondents to the questionnaire are requested to simply affirm or deny items with reference to their perceived health state on the day of completion.

The FLP is similar to the SIP but is a slightly modified version designed specifically for use in England. Amendments were made to the wording and weight values of some items.[13] The changes in wording were intended to make the questionnaire acceptable and easily understandable to English respondents. After rewording some of the items the weighting exercise undertaken for the original questionnaire was then repeated and minor amendments made to weights attached to a small number of the items. These changes are intended to reflect British rather than American valuations of the effect of certain states of subjective ill health upon well-being. The differences are quite minor, but the FLP is recommended over the original SIP for use on British populations and samples. The FLP, like its American counterpart, is one of the longer generic health measures but despite this, has gained widespread use and has become something of a 'gold standard' by which other measures tend to be judged.[3]

The FLP is a measure of sickness-related behavioural dysfunction as assessed by an individual's perception of the effect of illness upon usual daily activities. The profile contains 12 dimensions that ill health may adversely affect. These are ambulation, body care and movement, mobility, household management, recreation and pastimes, social interaction, emotion, alertness, sleep and rest, eating, communication and work. Table 4.1 provides examples of items on the 12 dimensions of the FLP. Respondents answer either 'Yes' or 'No' to items and can gain a score from 0 to 100 on each of the dimensions except work where the score range is from 0 to 70. As noted above, each item carries a specific weight ascribed to it by the designers, with higher values indicating worse health state relative to other items. Except for the work category, it is possible for respondents to affirm all or none of the questions on a particular category. This is not possible with the work dimension as one of the items asks respondents whether they have retired or are not presently working due to ill health, whilst the remainder ask about the influence of health problems upon ability to perform work: obviously one cannot be both presently not working and also having trouble at work due to health problems. A single figure can be generated from the measure, as can a summary physical score and psychosocial score, although these are less frequently reported and only limited research has been undertaken to determine how meaningful are the results from these summary indices.

In total there are 136 items on the FLP but due to the amount of time required to complete all the sections, it is not uncommon for researchers to select a number of categories from the questionnaire rather than administering the entire instrument. However, this does have the disadvantage of not enabling researchers to calculate the overall index score of ill health, which can only be done when the entire instrument is used. Furthermore, the physical summary score (gained by summing the categories of ambulation, body care and movement, mobility and household management) and the psychosocial summary score (gained

Dimension	Item content (example)
Ambulation	I only walk with help from someone else
Body care and movement	I stay lying down most of the time
Mobility	I stay in one room
Household management	I do not do heavy work around the house
Recreation and pastimes	I go out less often to enjoy myself
Emotion	I talk hopelessly about the future
Social interaction	I go out less often to visit people
Alertness	I make more mistakes than usual
Sleep and rest	I sit for much of the day
Eating	I eat much less than usual
Communication	I do not speak clearly when I am under stress
Work	I am not getting as much work done as usual

Table 4.1 FLP domains and example items. This table is for guidance only and does not contain the entire FLP, so should not be used in this form.

by summing the categories of recreation and pastimes, social interaction, emotion, alertness and sleep and rest) can only be calculated if the appropriate dimensions are included. It is important to note that perhaps the greatest difference between the original SIP and the FLP is the calculation of these two summary scales, as the SIP requires different dimensions to be summed to gain scores for the 'physical' and 'psychosocial' dimensions. For this reason results from studies utilizing the SIP are not fully comparable to those using the FLP on these two summary scores. Researchers must be sure that they are calculating these scores appropriately and not using the scoring system of the FLP on the SIP or vice versa. Intending users should consult appropriate reference books.[3,4]

The SIP/FLP has been recommended for use by self-completion, telephone administration or face-to-face interviewer administration. However, the questionnaire is substantially longer than many other health status questionnaires (it is over three times longer than any of the other instruments reviewed in this publication) and can take substantial periods of time to complete (up to 30 minutes). The length of the measure can adversely affect response rates, especially in postal surveys and where the inclusion of a health status questionnaire is supplemental to detailed questioning in other areas (for example, in a health and lifestyle survey). Whilst shorter form versions of the SIP have been developed little work has been undertaken to validate them and to date, they have gained only limited use.

The SIP and FLP have been subject to extensive trials of reliability and validity. Results have been encouraging, with the questionnaire revealing high levels of internal consistency and test-retest reliability.[5,6,13] Less work has been done on the sensitivity to change, or 'responsiveness', of the questionnaire. This is an important feature of health status questionnaires, especially when utilized in studies to evaluate the efficacy of treatments. It has been suggested that the questionnaire does lack measurement sensitivity,[14] although one study indicated it to be as good or better than other instruments in the detection of change.[15] Subsequent research has shown that the sensitivity of the questionnaire varies according to dimensions selected. In a study of the use of the FLP in arthritis patients, the questionnaire indicated, for example, very little change over three months on the household management items, whilst a moderate change was indicated on the social dimension. This study compared a number of health measures, none of which gave consistent indications of change on all dimensions.[16] Furthermore, it has been suggested that results on the questionnaire may be influenced by place of completion. It has been noted that many items on the mobility dimension may be affirmed by inpatients because they are in hospital, but not because they are functionally incapable.[17] For example, patients may affirm the item 'I stay in bed more' not necessarily because of ill health but because they are in hospital. Obviously, cautious interpretation of results from the FLP/SIP is needed when patients have completed the questionnaire initially as inpatients and are then followed up as outpatients.

Despite the claim that the instrument is comprehensive it contains no dimension specifically aimed at the assessment of pain. It is one of the few questionnaires lacking this dimension, which has been cited as a central dimension in the assessment of health state and an important area for health status questionnaires to cover.[18] Furthermore, wording of some of the items of the questionnaire is ambiguous. For example, the SIP/FLP requests respondents to complete the questionnaire with reference to today. They are thus asked to affirm or deny items on the basis of how they are feeling today. The basis of this judgement should, further, be related to their health. Let us take the example outlined in the SIP/FLP itself. It concerns the ability to drive. The statement given is 'I am not driving my car'. Thus, if a respondent cannot drive a car today and this is due to a health complaint, then they should affirm the question 'I am not driving my car'. If they are not driving because they never learnt to do so, then they must answer this question in the negative. Thus, respondents are asked to make two judgements for each response. It could be argued that in such a long questionnaire (136 items) respondents may well forget or ignore the initial rubric. However, even if this were not the case, some questions don't make any sense on the basis of the rubric. For example, for the item 'I have attempted suicide', respondents must tick 'Yes' or 'No' to this item in relation to *today*. Further, they must not tick 'Yes' if they have attempted suicide today but did so because their spouse has been killed in a car accident (this is, after all, not a problem with *their* health). Maybe it would be legitimate to tick 'Yes' if the respondent reasoned that their mental health had been adversely affected by a relative's death and they had attempted suicide today!

Such ambiguous and potentially meaningless questions can lead to respondents not completing all the questions or, indeed, the whole questionnaire. Nonetheless, the FLP remains one of the best established measures in the field, is made freely available for use both in research and medical evaluation and assessment and, unlike many other multidimensional questionnaires, can provide an overall figure of health state. It has been used in surveys of the disabled, in randomized controlled trials and in a very wide variety of conditions such as chronic obstructive airways disease, migraine, rheumatoid arthritis, endstage renal disease, low back pain and Parkinson's disease. Whilst incorporation into day-to-day clinical practice seems an unlikely use for such a long questionnaire, it remains a serious contender for those considering measuring health state in randomized control trials, clinical trials and research.

The Nottingham Health Profile (NHP)

Perhaps the most widely used instrument designed in Britain is the Nottingham Health Profile (NHP).[7,8] The originators of this profile argued that despite numerous attempts to develop measures of self-assessed health, no instrument had been designed that was short, easy to complete and generic. They remarked that:

There are a number of criticisms that can be made of existing measures . . . although not all of the following comments apply to each instrument. First, they are often long and complicated with ambiguous statements; second, scoring and weighting for seriousness often reflect the values of the physician not those of the lay person; thirdly, the focus of the measures may be on too narrow an area, for example disability; and fourthly, where the answers are summed to a single score or index this can be derived in many different ways and involve the addition of scores not logically related.[7]

The Nottingham Health Profile was designed to overcome such problems.

Work on the measure began in the late 1970s. Preliminary work outlined the sort of structure and contents of the NHP and the final questionnaire was published in the mid 1980s.[7,8] The measure contained two sections, of which the first, containing 38 items, is intended to measure perceptions of subjective health on six different dimensions which ill health may adversely affect. The items are distributed between the areas of pain, physical mobility, emotional reactions, sleep disturbance, social isolation and energy. Each item carries a specific weight, ascribed to it by the originators from a weighting technique they refer to as Thurstone's method of paired comparisons.[19] Questions were generated for the questionnaire by interviewing lay people and clinicians and weights assigned by assessments of the relative severity of the statements by similar groups. The method of assigning weights to the items is described fully elsewhere,[7,8,19] but these weights are intended to reflect the relative seriousness of items on the questionnaire. Respondents answer 'Yes' or 'No' to the questions and can affirm any number of the items on the NHP which they believe reflect their health state 'at the moment'. Scores range from 0 (indicating good health) to 100 (indicating poor health).

The developers of the NHP decided it should tap only the severe end of ill health and so items which reflected minor health problems were discarded. They suggest that the restriction to items which represent severe problems was necessary to avoid picking up large numbers of false positives. This reflects the original intention of the developers which was to design an instrument for use in population surveys which could be employed in planning health service provision.[7,8] The developers have subsequently attempted to distance themselves from their original position[20] and claim that the NHP is essentially a tool for assessing perceived ill health amongst the chronically ill and evaluating the efficacy of medical interventions upon subjective health. An example of items to be found on the NHP is shown in Table 4.2.

Substantial work has gone into validating the NHP and ensuring its reliability over time.[21] It has been tested for face, content and criterion validity.

The NHP has been utilized extensively – for example, in studies of the general population, on unemployed and re-employed men, on pregnant women and on patients with migraine, osteoarthritis and rheumatoid arthritis, in studies of cholecystectomy, heart/lung transplants and clinical trials of antihypertensive medication. A substantial number of projects which have utilized the NHP are summarized in Hunt et al.[22] Data suggest that the measure is good at identifying people with chronic illnesses and distinguishing between different conditions. Furthermore,

Dimension	Item content (example)
Energy	I'm tired all the time
Pain	I find it painful to change position
Emotional reactions	I wake up feeling depressed
Sleep	I sleep badly at night
Social isolation	I feel I am a burden to people
Physical mobility	I'm unable to walk at all

Table 4.2 NHP domains and example items. This table is for guidance only and does not contain the entire NHP, so cannot be used in this form.

more recent work with the profile has suggested that the questionnaire can be scored in such a way as to gain a single-index figure. This procedure requires the removal of certain items from the original 38 in the questionnaire. The revised scoring gives a 'distress' score. The questionnaire can be administered in this 24-item shortened format in order to gain a single-index figure of health-related distress, which can be used in QALY-type cost utility analysis.[23] However, the distress score has been relatively infrequently used.

A number of translated versions exist which can permit the use of the instrument in crosscultural trials. The instrument is short and easy to complete. However, as with all measurement tools, it has limitations. The decision of the developers to tap only the severe end of ill health means that data gained from the questionnaire tend to be highly skewed, with most respondents gaining zero or low scores on many or, indeed, all the dimensions of the profile.[24] Due to this 'floor effect', the NHP may not always be an appropriate tool in the assessment of change over time. For example, respondents may gain zero scores at time 1 ('baseline') but, despite an improvement by time 2 ('follow-up'), such change is not detected. Further problems with the NHP have been mentioned elsewhere. It has, for example, been noted that the dimensions of pain and mobility are confounded,[25] that the method of weighting the severity of items leads to illogical and incoherent results[26] and despite the attempts of the developers to produce an instrument that was simple to understand and easy and quick to complete, other measures have been found to have a higher response rate in community surveys.[27] Indeed, Donovan et al.[28] have highlighted the difficulties many respondents have in completing the NHP as the 'Yes/No' dichotomy can prevent people expressing how they really feel.

The Dartmouth COOP Charts

The Dartmouth COOP Charts were developed by the Dartmouth Primary Care Co-operative Information Project (the COOP Project), a collaborative research network of primary care clinicians, in affiliation with the Department of Community and Family Medicine at Dartmouth Medical School in America. Aware of the need for practical solutions to the problem of assessing patients' functional status, the group of researchers set out to design a set of simple measures that would not only fulfil requirements of accuracy, validity and reliability, but would also be simple and quick to complete and that could be scored by clinicians without the need for sophisticated scoring algorithms.

The COOP Chart system was based upon the following six premises:[9]

- The questionnaire should produce reliable and valid results on a core set of dimensions of function and well-being.

- The questionnaire should be acceptable to patients, physicians and other medical staff.

- The questionnaire should be applicable to a wide range of problems and diagnoses.

- The questionnaire should possess a high degree of face validity.

- The questionnaire should produce easily interpretable scores.

- The questionnaire should provide clinically useful information.

The COOP system consists of nine charts which measure physical, social and role functioning, emotional status, social support, pain, quality of life, overall health and health change.

The COOP Charts are similar in their simplicity to Snellen charts used to measure visual acuity. Each chart, which is typically typed onto a sheet of card 11 × 8.5 inches or, in the UK, on to A4, poses a simply worded question regarding the patient's status on the relevant dimension over the past four weeks. There are five response categories to each question, with each response category being linked to a drawing intended to represent the health state. Two of the charts are reproduced in Figure 4.1. The COOP Charts are reproduced in full elsewhere.[9, 29]

Unlike the NHP, FLP and SF-36 (for information on the latter see below), the Dartmouth COOP Charts were developed specifically for use in clinical practice and, most specifically, in primary care.[9, 10] The charts

DAILY ACTIVITIES

During the past 4 weeks . . .
How much difficulty have you had doing your usual activities or task, both inside and outside the house because of your physical and emotional health?

No difficulty at all	1
A little bit of difficulty	2
Some difficulty	3
Much difficulty	4
Could not do	5

SOCIAL ACTIVITIES

During the past four weeks . . .
Has your physical and emotional health limited your social activities with family, friends, neighbours or groups?

Not at all	1
Slightly	2
Moderately	3
Quite a bit	4
Extremely	5

Figure 4.1 Examples of the Dartmouth COOP Charts. (Copyright © Trustees of Dartmouth College COOP Project; support provided by the Henry J Kaiser Family Foundation.)

were initially developed with the intention of providing primary care clinicians with an efficient measurement tool for assessing and monitoring patient function in routine practice.[30] The content of each chart was derived from expert advice from clinicians and health measurement professionals. Furthermore, the charts went through a number of iterations before taking on their current form.

The charts can be administered by self-completion or the provider (nurse, doctor, physiotherapist, etc.) can administer them. Each chart takes between 30 and 45 seconds to complete and so the entire group can be completed in about five minutes. As there are no complex scoring algorithms results from the charts can be written down immediately into patient notes. The designers do not advocate summing the responses to gain a single-index figure of health status.

The COOP Charts have been assessed for reliability and validity. They have been shown to have high levels of test-retest reliability, although elderly patients and those in lower socioeconomic classes gain less consistent results.[9] Furthermore, when compared with longer measures of health status, the COOP Charts have compared well. Whilst the instrument could not be expected to have the same degree of precision as longer measures, the results do suggest the charts tap similar information.[10] However, with any measure that uses single items to tap dimensions of health, there is inevitably compromise in reliability.

It has been suggested that the charts improve doctor–patient communication and can influence patient management. According to the Dartmouth COOP Project, clinicians claim that the charts improve communication with patients, provide a clearer picture of the functional status of the patient and can modify treatment plans. Similarly, patients enjoy completing the charts and report that the exercise influenced communication with their physician, provided important information and played a useful part in their treatment.[31]

The charts were not developed for use in samples and populations, although there is evidence to suggest that they can be used in this manner. The primary purpose of the COOP Project was to design a measure that would be of use in routine clinical practice. Thus, when undertaking evaluations of medical interventions, for example in randomized controlled trials, the charts may not always be the most appropriate health status measure. Furthermore, the designers themselves have suggested that the content and style of the pictures may influence patient response and further research needs to be undertaken to determine the extent of this upon results. Nonetheless, the charts have been widely used in America although they are still used relatively infrequently in Britain. However, as an adjunct to the clinical interview and as a general indication of patient health status in populations, this instrument is certainly worthy of consideration.

The SF-20, SF-36 and related measures

The SF-36 was one of the products of the RAND Corporation's Health Insurance Experiment (HIE) and subsequent Medical Outcomes Study (MOS). The Health Insurance Experiment and the Medical Outcomes Study long-form general health surveys were the precursors of the short-form instruments. The distinctive feature of both studies was the decision to collect patient-assessed outcome measures as well as traditional clinical and laboratory measures of health and illness.

The RAND HIE was a US federal government-funded study which ran between 1974 and 1982 to examine the effect of health payment systems on the use of health services. Approximately 4000 people aged 14 to 61, representative of the general population of the area where they lived,[32] were enrolled into the study from six sites. Participants were followed for three years, 30% of whom were followed up for a further two years. One of the major findings of the study was that those enrolled in a co-payment scheme made a third fewer medical visits and were hospitalized a third less often than those receiving care free at the point of entry. To determine whether those receiving 'free' care were healthier as a result, measures were developed to evaluate the effect of cost sharing on health status. These measures included instruments to assess subjective health. The HIE health questionnaire contained 108 items which were administered at entry and on leaving the study. Self-assessed general health was measured on five dimensions: physical functioning, role functioning, mental health, social contacts and health perceptions. Results led to two main conclusions: that free care did not improve health status regardless of how it was measured and that the HIE clearly demonstrated the potential of scales constructed from self-administered surveys as reliable and valid tools for assessing changes in health status for both adults and children in the general population. The HIE health questionnaire consequently provided the background for the Medical Outcomes Study (MOS) patient-assessed health measures.

The MOS was a two-year prospective study with two major aims: first, to determine whether variations in patient outcomes could be explained by variations in system of care, clinician speciality and clinician's technical and interpersonal style, and second, to develop instruments for the routine monitoring of patient outcomes in medical practice, specifically self-administered questionnaires and generic scales.[33]

Random samples of physicians were drawn from different health care settings in Boston, Chicago, and Los Angeles. Over 22 000 patients who consulted the sampled doctors during nine-day screening periods between February and November 1986 completed a form in which they evaluated their health status and treatment. Of these, over 3000 patients with one or more of a number of specific health problems or 'tracer' conditions, including diabetes mellitus, hypertension, heart disease and depression, were selected for the longitudinal study. Over the following two years hospitalizations and treatments were monitored and the health status of these patients was repeatedly measured. The study was then able to correlate the structures (e.g. the method of payment), the processes (e.g. the clinician's interpersonal style) and the outcomes (both clinical/laboratory measures and patient assessed) of medical treatment.

The largest set of MOS health measures included in a single questionnaire, the MOS Functioning and Well-Being (MOSFWB) Profile, was administered in the baseline Patient Assessment Questionnaire (PAQ) to patients who were identified as having one or more tracer conditions. These patients were asked to complete the profile at the start of the longitudinal phase of the study. This measure is recommended for studies in which the 'full set' of MOS scales is required. It includes 35 scales and 149 items measuring physical and role functioning, social, family and sexual functioning, mobility, psychological distress/well-being, cognitive functioning, health perceptions, health distress, energy/fatigue, sleep, pain and symptoms. Due to the length and breadth of this profile, completion takes an estimated 30–37 minutes. The full PAQ, including the MOSFWB Profile, amounts to 245 items. Consequently, short-form measures have been developed which require less time to complete.

The Short Form 20 general health survey (SF-20) was developed within the MOS in the quest for a generic health status measure which could satisfy a number of potentially conflicting criteria. Ideally, the authors wished to develop a measure which was short enough to be completed quickly yet was also comprehensive (covering as many dimensions of health as possible) with psychometrically sound, multi-item scales.[34] Part of the rationale behind the pursuit of short-form health status measures was the idea of 'outcomes management' whereby clinical, financial and health outcomes data could form a national database with which to inform decision making. In this schema, patient-generated outcomes data are then elicited from short-form subjective health status instruments. Within the MOS the aim was to develop and refine the SF-20 as a method for assessing functional status and well-being while at the same time examining its sensitivity, as a generic measure, to the impact of disease and treatments.

The HIE provided the basis for the 20 item short-form instrument. Eighteen items were drawn from the parent instrument. The remaining items were single-item measures of social functioning and bodily pain which were developed following experience with the similar measures in the HIE. Items on the questionnaire were completed on a 'Likert'-type response format (with answers to questions from choices such as 'Limited a lot', 'Limited a little', 'Not limited at all', rather than on weighted dichotomous 'Yes'/'No' scales, as is the case in the Nottingham Health Profile and FLP/Sickness Impact Profile, outlined above). Like any health status measure, the SF-20 is required to fulfil a number of criteria if it is to be of value. A measure should be:

• appropriate for the research issue in terms of the content and dimensions of health and the levels of health or ill health it covers

• reliable

• valid

• practically useful

• sensitive to change.

An examination of the extent to which the SF-20 fulfils the above criteria helps to highlight the shortcomings of the instrument and hence the decision to supersede it with the SF-36.

One of the aims of the MOS was to develop a measure which would be appropriate to general population groups as well as to patient groups. The MOS instruments are described as 'generic', in that they are intended to assess health concepts that represent basic human values relevant to everyone's health status and well-being regardless of age, disease or treatment group. The SF-20 has been used in a variety of general population and patient groups. Seventeen of the core 18 items drawn from the HIE questionnaire were included in a telephone interview study conducted by Louis Harris Associates in 1984, involving 2000 adults in US households half of whom were enrolled in health maintenance organizations (HMOs) and half in fee for service (FFS) systems. The results provided a general population sample with which patient samples from the MOS could be compared. In the Medical Outcomes Study all 20 items of the instrument were administered to a randomly selected half of the total screening sample totalling approximately 11 000 adults. This provided a substantial dataset on which to assess the reliability and validity of the measure. The internal consistency of the SF-20 has been examined in a variety of patient group samples. Internal consistency indicates the homogeneity of the items of a scale and is measured by the degree to which they correlate with each other and with the overall score. On the SF-20 two health dimensions, bodily pain and social functioning, are measured by single items which clearly prohibits this type of reliability measurement. On the other four multi-item scales, reliability coefficients ranged from 0.76 upwards. This was lower, but not much lower, than those gained for the full-length long-form parent profiles. Reliabilities at this level satisfy the minimum requirements for group assessment.

Whilst results indicated that the SF-20 had high levels of internal reliability consistency on multi-item domains, social functioning and pain were single-item measures and hence could not be evaluated for internal reliability consistency. Indeed, Ware has suggested that ideally domains should contain multiple items,[35] so the decision to include domains measured with single items seems uncharacteristic and was indeed one of the grounds for the development of an improved short-form health survey instrument. Furthermore, the SF-20 was shown to manifest a 'floor effect' when administered to seriously ill patients.[36] The SF-36 was an attempt to overcome these problems.

The SF-36 is perhaps the most famous questionnaire developed from the HIE and MOS. The instrument contains eight dimensions and a single item requesting information as to perceived health change over the past year. The dimensions, and number of items per dimension in the questionnaire, are:

- physical functioning (ten items)
- role limitations due to physical problems (four items)
- role limitations due to emotional problems (three items)
- social functioning (two items)
- mental health (five items)
- energy/vitality (four items)
- pain (two items)
- general health perception (five items).

Some of the items on the questionnaire are reproduced in Figure 4.2. Scores on each of the domains are gained by summing item responses and, with the use of a scoring algorithm, transforming these raw scores onto a scale from 0 (for poor health) to 100 (good health). This, it should be noted, is the opposite to the scoring rules of the FLP/SIP and NHP, where 0 indicates good health and 100 poor health. The developers suggest that the SF-36 should take respondents approximately five to ten minutes to complete and evidence from its use in the UK suggests that respondents find it easy to complete, as response rates in postal surveys using the questionnaire are high.[37]

Validity testing of the SF-36 has been carried out in the US and the UK and has included examination of the content, criterion and construct validity of the instrument.

One of the aims of the SF-36 was to improve the content validity of the short-form measures compared to the 20-item scale. To achieve this, the number of health dimensions was increased to eight and the number of items almost doubled to 36. In terms of the validity of the scales it is worth briefly describing how each was developed and modified from the SF-20 version. The two single-item scales, social functioning and bodily pain, were developed into multi-item versions.

Social functioning

The social functioning dimension was expanded to a two-item scale in the SF-36, tapping two types of health-related effects on social functioning: the extent to which physical or emotional health problems limit interaction with others, and the changes in usual levels of social activity due to changes in health. The MOS developed their own set of four questions on social functioning for the MOSFWB Profile, two of which were utilized in the SF-36.

Bodily pain

The SF-20 asks about the intensity of bodily pain, whereas the SF-36 also asks about the degree to which pain interferes with normal functional abilities. These two items were drawn from the 12–item pain battery in the MOSFWB Profile which in turn was adapted from the Wisconsin Brief Pain Questionnaire.[38]

Multi-item scales in the SF-20 were also modified for the SF-36.

Physical functioning

The physical functioning scale used in the SF-20 was composed of six items covering seven levels of physical functioning. For the SF-36 the measure was increased to the full long-form ten-item scale covering 21

In general, would you say your health is (*please tick* **one** *box*)

Excellent	Very good	Good	Fair	Poor
☐	☐	☐	☐	☐

HEALTH AND DAILY ACTIVITIES

The following questions are about activities you might do during a typical day. Does your health limit you in these activities? If so, how much? (*Please tick* **one** *box on each line*)

	Yes, limited a lot	Yes, limited a little	No, not limited at all
(a) **Moderate activities**, such as moving a table, pushing a vacuum, bowling or playing golf	☐	☐	☐
(b) Climbing **several** flights of stairs	☐	☐	☐

During the **past 4 weeks**, have you had any of the following problems with your work or other regular daily activities **as a result of your physical health**? (*Please answer* **Yes** *or* **No** *to each question*)

	Yes	No
(a) **Accomplished less** than you would like	☐	☐
(b) Were limited in the **kind** of work or other activities	☐	☐

During the **past 4 weeks** how much did **pain** interfere with your normal work (including work both outside the home and housework)? (*Please tick* **one** *box*)

Not at all	A little bit	Moderately	Quite a bit	Extremely
☐	☐	☐	☐	☐

These questions are about how you feel and how things have been with you **during the past month**. For each question, please indicate the one answer that comes closest to the way you have been feeling. (*Please tick* **one** *box on each line*)

How much time during **the last month:**	All of the time	Most of the time	A good bit of the time	Some of the time	A little of the time	None of the time
(a) Have you felt calm and peaceful?	☐	☐	☐	☐	☐	☐
(b) Did you have a lot of energy?	☐	☐	☐	☐	☐	☐

Figure 4.2 Example items for the SF-36 and SF-12. This figure is for guidance only and does not contain the entire SF-36/SF-12, so should not be used in this form.

levels, making detection of small differences in function possible. Items were adapted from 'nine existing measures of physical functioning'. The MOSFWB Profile is composed of three physical functioning measures: a ten-item physical functioning scale, a single-item satisfaction with physical ability measure and a two-item mobility measure. Although the authors recommend using all three measures together,[39] the SF-36 contains only the ten-item scale.

Role functioning

For the SF-20, a two-item scale was taken from the HIE role functioning scale. As this proved to be a rather coarse scale a number of changes were made for the SF-36. The role functioning dimension was expanded into two in order to capture role limitations due to physical health (four items) and emotional health (three items). New scales were created following a pilot study using items from published questionnaires and additional open-ended questions.

Mental health

The basis for the MOSFWB Profile was the Mental Health Inventory developed for the HIE composed of 38 items. A five-item version was constructed from those questions in the Mental Health Inventory which best predicted the summary score for the 38-item set. This shortened version was utilized in the SF-20 and was retained unchanged in the SF-36.

Energy/vitality

A four-item scale of vitality (energy level and fatigue) was added to the SF-36, a dimension of health not included in the SF-20. As with the mental health dimension, items were drawn from the Mental Health Inventory fielded in the HIE.

General health perceptions

The five-item current health subscale of the 26-item Health Perceptions Questionnaire (HPQ) utilized in the HIE was also used for the SF-20. It was decided to use a more comprehensive sample of items from the HPQ for the SF-36. Instead, five items from the General Health Rating Index (GHRI), itself developed from the HPQ, were used.

Change in health

A single item measuring change in health in the previous year was also included in the SF-36, although this item is not used to score any of the health dimensions.

A broad indication as to the meaning of scores on the SF-36 is provided in Table 3.1.

The MOS researchers undertook criterion validation of each scale on the SF-36. The criterion for each scale of the SF-36 was the full length MOS parent version. Results suggested the SF-36 stood up well against the longer form measures. Within the UK, criterion validity of the SF-36 has been examined in data gained from the Oxford Healthy Life Survey, a large-scale survey of a randomly selected group of respondents living in Northamptonshire, Buckinghamshire, Berkshire and Oxfordshire. The general health perceptions item, asking people to define their health in general from 'excellent' through to 'poor', was used as the criterion against which the other items were tested. Although it is not common practice to use an item from a questionnaire to evaluate the criterion validity of that measure, the item is one which has been used in other studies to evaluate the validity of other instruments and, moreover, the item contributes to only one dimension and therefore does not contribute to the scale scores for the other seven dimensions. Results from this analysis provide evidence for the criterion validity of the instrument on a general population sample.[40]

Construct validity of the SF-36 has been measured by comparing scores with hypothesized score distributions. As expected, men, higher social classes, younger age groups, those without chronic illness and those who had not consulted their general practitioner within the last two weeks scored higher than others, indicating better health.[27] In order to assess convergent and discriminant validity, Brazier and colleagues compared the SF-36 with the Nottingham Health Profile. Comparable dimensions of the two instruments generally correlated well (with the exception of the items measuring social functioning/isolation which were each addressing different aspects of social well-being) while item to own scale correlation was higher than item to other scale correlation.[27] In the United States, the SF-36 has undergone validity testing within the MOS using both psychometric and clinical criteria. Psychometric criteria were used to assess the extent to which each of the eight dimensions was an indicator of the two major, underlying concepts of physical health and mental health.[41] This was done by measuring the validity of each scale and comparing it to the 'most valid scale' for that dimension, that is, the scale which shared the most variance with either the physical or mental component of health.[41] By doing so, it was possible to estimate the degree to which a scale was a valid measure of physical and/or mental health status. Validity was also measured using clinical criteria: in order to investigate hypothesized relationships between patients, the SF-36 was administered to four patient groups each differing in physical and/or mental health status. It was expected that scales measuring physical health (i.e. physical functioning, role limitations due to physical health, and bodily pain) would be most valid in distinguishing between groups differing in severity of chronic medical conditions, while scales measuring general mental health (i.e. the mental health scale and role limitations due to emotional problems) would be most valid in distinguishing between groups differing in the presence and severity of psychiatric disorders. Results indicated that both psychometric and clinical tests provided consistent information about the underlying nature of each scale and the degree to which each scale measured that component.

The internal reliability consistency of items in the eight dimensions of the SF-36 has been tested in a number of applications and reported in both the US and the UK. In the latter, internal reliability consistency estimates have been calculated for general population groups and items within dimensions have been found to be highly correlated,[27] indicating that the items of each dimension are tapping a single underlying attribute.

Applications and recent developments of the Short-Form Measures

Measures resulting from the Medical Outcomes Study and the Health Insurance Programme have been used extensively in America and are gaining increasingly widespread use in England. The SF-20 and SF-36 have been applied to population samples and in the Medical Outcomes Study, to patients with hypertension, diabetes, arthritis, back problems and myocardial infarction, amongst many others. Within the United Kingdom many studies have utilized the measures in population surveys and in a wide variety of groups including, for example, patients presenting with hernia, menorrhagia, low back pain, Parkinson's disease, heart attack, hypertension, arthritis, depression, diabetes and urinary tract symptoms. An annotated bibliography has been published to help users locate publications appropriate to the client group under investigation.[42] It is worth noting that the SF-36 has been translated into a number of different languages and validated in countries other than North America and the United Kingdom. Further information on the crosscultural adaptation of the instrument undertaken by the International Quality of Life Assessment (IQOLA) project members is detailed elsewhere.[43]

The SF-36 is the product of a substantial amount of development work undertaken in America. It is short and covers a wide range of areas that may be adversely affected by illness. It contains items that are less severe than those found on the NHP and, as such, has been found to be more sensitive to lower levels of disability.[27] Population norms are available for use in the British context.[37] Response rates in random samples using the questionnaire have been shown to be high.[27,37] The questionnaire was designed to supplement disease-specific measures when used on samples of patients. This should be borne in mind by those who intend to use the questionnaire to evaluate treatment regimes. Indeed, the appropriateness of the measure for the elderly and some patient groups has been questioned.[44] Those who are unsure of the appropriateness of the measure for a particular sample or population would be wise to pilot it before use in the main study. Furthermore, no single-index figure of health status can, as yet, be gained from any of the short-form measures, although work is underway in the UK to develop methods of aggregating the data from the SF-36 into an index figure.

However, two summary scores measuring emotional health and physical health can be derived from the measure.[45] T is was achieved by undertaking a higher order factor analysis of the eight dimensions of the SF-36. This led to a two-factor solution, which reflects two aspects of health status, namely physical functioning and mental health. Consequently it is possible to score the SF-36 to gain the eight-dimension scores and/or to score it to get the two summary scores, which are entitled the physical component summary (PCS) and the mental health component summary (MCS). The statistical procedures which need to be undertaken to produce the summary scores are documented in a user manual.[46] The advantage of the summary scores is that they summarize a great deal of information in two relatively simple scores. This not only aids interpretation but also reduces the likelihood of chance statistical findings due to multiple comparisons.

The procedures used by the SF-36 developers have been undertaken in the UK and produce remarkably similar results.[47] Indeed, results gained from using the UK algorithms to calculate the PCS and MCS are correlated with the US results at the astonishing level of 0.99! This may provide some support for simply using the US algorithms with datasets in both the UK and US as this seems the most economical and, for that matter, simple approach to constructing these measures. In any case, the summary scores are standardized to a mean of 50 and standard deviation of 10 (this is known as a standardized score). Thus, scores on either the PCS or MCS which fall below 50 are below the average for the population whilst those above 50 are above the average. Consequently it is possible to interpret PCS/MCS scores in the light of published norms. For example, one study showed that patients with sleep apnoea indicated very poor health prior to treatment, with a large proportion of patients gaining scores that would place them in the bottom third of the population. After treatment a large proportion of the patients gained scores in the top 50% of population scores. Such norm-based interpretation gives users a sense of the state of health of patients, in relation to the general population, before and after treatment.[48]

Recently a 12-item health survey has been introduced,[49] which produces scores for eight dimensions (the same as those on the SF-36) as well as the two summary measures of health status (the physical and emotional summary scores). The measure was designed for users who essentially wish to tap the latter summary aspects of subjective health status. The eight-dimension scores yield less precise scores than the SF-36. The SF-12 is useful in studies where a short yet valid and reliable health status measure is required. Comparison of scores on the summary scores derived from the SF-36 and SF-12 indicate that the shorter version mirrors the results of the longer form with considerable accuracy.

Criticism of the SF-36 has been forthcoming, with perhaps the most common problems reported being those of ambiguity in some of the wording (one item contains an unhelpful double negative) and floor and ceiling effects being present in some of the eight dimensions (notably the two role performance scales). Recent work has led to an updated version of the SF-36 which has improved wording and standardized response categories which will lead to improved precision and sensitivity and will reduce floor and ceiling effects. The measure, the SF-36 Version 2, has been used relatively infrequently to date but is likely to become the standard version of the SF-36 in the future.[50, 51]

Summary

This chapter has outlined the development and application of the most widely used measures of general health available. It highlights some of the difficulties involved in creating what, on the face of it, would seem to be a relatively simple thing – a questionnaire that assesses health. Those considering using general measures of health should be familiar with the measures discussed, in terms of their development, testing and application.

References

1 Bowling A (1997) *Measuring Health: a review of quality of life measurement scales*, 2nd edn. Open University Press, Buckingham.

2 Bowling A (1995) *Measuring Disease: a review of disease-specific quality of life measurement scales*. Open University Press, Buckingham.

3 McDowell I, Newell C (1996) *Measuring Health: a guide to rating scales and questionnaires*. Oxford University Press, New York.

4 Wilkin D, Hallam L, Doggett M (1992) *Measures of Need and Outcome for Primary Health Care*. Oxford University Press, Oxford.

5 Bergner M, Bobbitt RA, Carter WB, Gilson BS (1981) The Sickness Impact Profile: development and final revision of a health status measure. *Medical Care*. **19**, 787–805.

6 Patrick D, Peach H (1989) *Disablement in the Community*. Oxford University Press, Oxford.

7 Hunt S, McEwen J, McKenna S (1985) Measuring health status: a new tool for clinicians and epidemiologists. *Journal of the Royal College of General Practitioners*. **35**: 185–8.

8 Hunt S, McEwen J, McKenna S (1986) *Measuring Health Status*. Croom Helm, Dover.

9 Beaufait DW, Nelson EC, Landgraf JM *et al.* (1992) COOP measures of functional status. In: *Tools for Primary Care Research: research methods for primary care, volume 2* (eds M Stewart, F Tudiver, MJ Bass, EV Dunn, PG Norton), Sage, London.

10 Nelson EC, Landgraf JM, Hays RD, Wasson JH, Kirk JW (1990) The functional status of patients: how can it be measured in physicians' offices? *Medical Care*. **28**: 1111–26.

11 Ware J, Sherbourne C (1992) The MOS 36–Item Short-Form Health Survey 1: conceptual framework and item selection. *Medical Care*. **30**: 473–83.

12 Ware JE, Kosinski M, Keller SD (1995) A 12 item short-form health survey. SF-12: scale construction and preliminary tests of reliability and validity. *Medical Care*. **34**: 220–33.

13 Patrick D, Sittampalam Y, Somerville S, Carter W, Bergner, M (1985) A cross cultural comparison of health status values. *American Journal of Public Health*. **71**: 1402–7.

14 Jette AM (1980) Health status indicators: their utility in chronic-disease evaluation research. *Journal of Chronic Diseases*. **33**: 567–79.

15 Liang MH, Fossel AH, Larson MG (1990) Comparisons of five health status instruments for orthopedic evaluation. *Medical Care.* **28**: 632–42.

16 Fitzpatrick R, Ziebland S, Jenkinson C, Mowat A, Mowat A (1992) The importance of sensitivity to change as a criterion for selection of health status measures. *Quality in Health Care.* **1**: 89–93.

17 Jenkinson C, Ziebland S, Fitzpatrick R, Mowat A, Mowat A (1991) Sensitivity to change of weighted and unweighted versions of two health status measures. *International Journal of Health Sciences.* **2**: 189–94.

18 Ware JE (1987) Standards for validating health measures: definition and content. *Journal of Chronic Diseases.* **40**: 473–80.

19 McKenna S, Hunt S, McEwen J (1981) Weighting the seriousness of perceived health problems using Thurstone's method of paired comparisons. *International Journal of Epidemiology.* **10**: 93–7.

20 Hunt S, McKenna S (1992) Validating the SF-36. *British Medical Journal.* **305**: 645.

21 McEwen J (1988) The Nottingham Health Profile. In: *Quality of Life: assessment and application* (eds SR Stewart, RM Rosser), MTP, Lancaster.

22 Hunt S, McKenna S (1991) *The Nottingham Health Profile User's Manual*, revised edn. Galen Research and Consultancy, Manchester.

23 McKenna S, Hunt S, Tennant A (1993) The development of a patient-completed index of distress from the Nottingham Health Profile: a new measure for use in cost-utility studies. *British Journal of Medical Economics.* **6**: 13–24.

24 Kind P, Carr-Hill R (1987) The Nottingham Health Profile: a useful tool for epidemiologists? *Social Science and Medicine.* **25**: 905–10.

25 Jenkinson C, Fitzpatrick R, Argyle M (1988) The Nottingham Health Profile: an analysis of its sensitivity in differentiating illness groups. *Social Science and Medicine.* **27**: 1411–14.

26 Jenkinson C (1991) Why are we weighting? A critical examination of the use of item weights in a health status measure. *Social Science and Medicine.* **32**: 1413–16.

27 Brazier JE, Harper R, Jones NMB *et al.* (1992) Validating the SF-36 Health Survey Questionnaire: new outcome measure for primary care. *British Medical Journal.* **305**: 160–4.

28 Donovan JL, Frankel SJ, Eyles JD (1993) Assessing the need for health status measures. *Journal of Epidemiology and Community Health.* **47**: 158–62.

29 Rowan K (1994) Global questions and scores. In: *Measuring Health and Medical Outcomes* (ed C Jenkinson), UCL Press, London.

30 Wasson J, Keller A, Rubenstein L, Hays R, Nelson E, Johnson D, and the Dartmouth Primary Care COOP Project (1992) Benefits and obstacles of health status assessment in ambulatory settings: the clinician's point of view. *Medical Care.* **30** (suppl): MS42–MS49.

31 Kraus N (1991) *The InterStudy Quality Edge,* **1**(1). InterStudy, Excelsior, Minneapolis.

32 Brook RH, Ware JE, Rogers WR *et al.* (1983) Does free care improve adults' health? Results from a randomised controlled trial. *New England Journal of Medicine.* **309**: 1426–34.

33 Tarlov AR, Ware JE, Greenfield S, Nelson EC, Perrin E, Zubkoff M (1989) The Medical Outcomes Study: an application of methods for monitoring the results of medical care. *Journal of the American Medical Association.* **262**: 925–30.

34 Stewart AL, Hays RD, Ware JE (1988) The MOS Short Form General Health Survey. *Medical Care.* **26**: 724–35.

35 Ware JE (1987) Standards for validating health measures: definition and content. *Journal of Chronic Diseases.* **40**: 473–80.

36 Bindman AB, Keane D, Lurie N (1990) Measuring health changes among severely ill patients: the floor phenomenon. *Medical Care.* **28**: 1142–52.

37 Jenkinson C, Coulter A, Wright L (1993) Short Form 36 (SF 36) Health Survey Questionnaire: normative data for adults of working age. *British Medical Journal.* **306**: 1437–40.

38 Daut RL, Cleeland CS, Flannery RC (1983) Development of the Wisconsin Brief Pain Questionnaire to assess pain in cancer and other diseases. *Pain.* **17**: 197–210.

39 Stewart AL, Kamberg CJ (1992) Physical functioning measures. In: *Measuring Functioning and Well Being: the Medical Outcomes Study approach* (eds AL Stewart, JE Ware), Duke University Press, London.

40 Jenkinson C, Wright L, Coulter A (1994) Criterion validity and reliability of the SF-36 in a population sample. *Quality of Life Research.* **3**: 7–12.

41 McHorney CA, Ware JE, Raczek AE (1993) The MOS 36-Item Short-Form Health Survey (SF-36): II. Psychometric and clinical tests of validity in measuring physical and mental health constructs. *Medical Care.* **31**: 247–63.

42 Shiely J-C, Bayliss MS, Keller SD, Tsai C, Ware JE (1996) *SF-36 Health Survey Annotated Bibliography (1988–1995).* The Health Institute, New England Medical Center, Boston. (Plus Supplement (1997).)

43 Aaronson NK, Acquadro C, Alonso J *et al.* (1992) International Quality of Life Assessment (IQOLA) Project. *Quality of Life Research.* **1**: 349–51.

44 Hayes V, Morris J, Wolfe C, Morgan M (1995) The SF-36 Health Survey Questionnaire: is it suitable for use with older adults? *Age and Ageing*. **24**: 120–5.

45 Ware JE, Kosinski M, Bayliss MS *et al.* (1995) Comparison of methods for scoring and statistical analysis of SF-36 health profile and summary measures: summary of results from the Medical Outcomes Study. *Medical Care*. **33**: AS264–AS279.

46 Ware JE, Kosinski M, Keller SD (1994) *SF-36 Physical and Mental Health Summary Scales: a user manual*. The Health Institute, New England Medical Center, Boston.

47 Jenkinson C, Layte R, Lawrence K (1997) Development and testing of the Medical Outcomes Study 36–item Short Form Health Survey Summary Scale Scores in the United Kingdom. *Medical Care*. **35**: 410–16.

48 Jenkinson C (1998) The SF-36 Physical and Mental Health Summary scores: a guide to interpretation. *Journal of Health Services Research and Policy*. **3**: 92–6.

49 Ware JE, Kosinski M, Keller SD (1995) A 12-item short-form health survey. Construction of scales and preliminary tests of reliability and validity. *Medical Care*. **34**: 220–33.

50 Ware JE, Kosinski M (1997) Improvements in the content and scoring of the SF-36 Health Survey. SF-36 site at http://www.sf-36.com/news/sf36-20.html.

51 Jenkinson C, Stewart-Brown S, Petersen S *et al.* (1998) Development and testing of the UK SF-36 Version II. *Journal of Epidemiology and Community Medicine*. In press.

5
Generic single-index measures of health status

Introduction

This chapter discusses two very different approaches to the evaluation of health status or quality of life which produce single indices. One approach requires social valuations of health status (i.e. asking large groups of people to assess the impact that adverse health states have on health-related quality of life) whilst the other asks individuals to select and value their own areas of health-related quality of life adversely affected by illness.

Single indices have advantages and disadvantages over profile measures of outcome. The first advantage, and perhaps the most obvious one, is that they appear to summarize a great deal of information in a simple single number. Second, and perhaps most controversially, some single indices can be used in cost-benefit analysis, which is undertaken by health economists and attempts to assess the benefits of treatment, taking into account the cost of the intervention. Such single indices must include social valuations of health states, an issue that will be covered below. However, some single-index measures are derived from simply summing up scores from a profile, are far too complex (i.e. provide too many health states which would take forever to value) or are derived from other psychometric techniques which do not provide social valuations and consequently are inappropriate for use in cost-benefit analysis.

This chapter considers not only measures designed for use in health economics but also measures that have been designed to measure individualized quality of life. The latter approach does not depend upon standardized questionnaires but upon respondents selecting the areas they individually think are important in their lives. Individualized measures are not appropriate for economic analyses but are, claim their supporters, able to reflect people's health-related quality of life accurately because the areas chosen are actually selected by each individual respondent. Such measures should, therefore, be highly responsive to any treatment which brings about changes in health.

Single-index measures in health economics

One of the main interests in health economics is to gain some insight into the value of treatment regimes in terms of both life-years gained (if appropriate) and subjective health status following treatment. Health status or quality of life measures used by economists are intended to reflect the utility of treatment. Utility, in this instance, refers to a subjective assessment of the well-being that is gained (or not!) from medical interventions.

The most common economic approach to the assessment of the value of medical interventions is to adjust the number of life-years gained from an intervention by the quality of life of those treated, a procedure that produces quality-adjusted life-years (QALYs). For example, if one assumes it is possible to measure health-related quality of life from 0 (worst possible state) to 1 (best possible state) and to be fairly certain of the number of years a person would live in a state then QALYs could be calculated. A person with perfect health (i.e. a score of 1) who was going to live ten years would gain ten QALYs (i.e. 1×10), whilst a person with only half-perfect health (0.5) who was going to live ten years would gain five QALYs (i.e. 0.5×10). The appeal of the QALY is that it enables evaluation of alternative programmes to be made on the basis of cost per QALY. One of the major challenges to this approach is how to successfully measure subjective health status or quality of life. Health status profiles, such as the SF-36 and FLP (discussed in Chapter 4), provide scores on a range of dimensions such as physical functioning, social interaction, pain, emotional functioning, mental health, etc. The primary purpose of such measures is not to give a single value for health status or quality of life. However, one of the limitations of multi-dimensional assessments is that comparison of outcomes between different conditions is difficult since different dimensions within the profile may assume varying degrees of significance according to the disease under consideration. Whilst these profiles permit comparison of health status for alternative treatments of the same condition, economic evaluation to determine resource allocation between conditions is not possible. Furthermore, whilst some profile measures can be summed to a single score that score is not based upon utility measurement, which is fundamental to the weighting of scores on the measures utilized in health economics. In order for economic analysis to be meaningful the quality of life needs to be expressed as a single index which could then be combined with measures of mortality to identify a QALY.

In order to incorporate utility measures into economic evaluations of health care, we must be able to rank medical outcomes in order of preference and establish the distance between positions on this scale, i.e. it is necessary to be able to determine how much better one outcome is than another. The three most commonly implemented approaches to this problem are magnitude estimation using a rating scale, time trade-off and the standard gamble.

Magnitude estimation requires subjects to place conditions on a continuum, for example between 0 and 100, which correspond to the least preferred and most preferred outcomes respectively. If a score of 100 represents perfect health, then a score of 50 would indicate that life in that condition would yield only half the utility enjoyed by someone who has no health problems. The same valuation could be secured by magnitude estimation techniques which ask respondents to state how much worse one condition is than another as a ratio.

The time trade-off approach asks respondents to identify a trade-off between a shorter life of perfect health and a longer life suffering from a chronic condition. Subjects are asked how many years of perfect health they would be willing to sacrifice in order to be relieved of the condition. A health state is valued by identifying the point at which an individual is indifferent between so many years of healthy life and a greater number of years of sickness. The ratio between these two determines the relevant quality of life score.

The standard gamble offers a choice between the certainty of continued life with a chronic condition or a gamble. There are two possible outcomes if the gamble of treatment is accepted: there is a probability p that perfect health will be restored, and probability $(1-p)$ that the patient will die. Respondents are asked to vary p until they are indifferent between taking the treatment gamble and continued suffering of the condition being valued. The value attributed to p represents the measure of utility attributed to that condition. The lower the score (i.e. the lower the probability of a cure which is regarded by the respondent as equivalent to continued existence in the poor health state), the lower the utility attached to that condition. Various projects have utilized these methods for gaining weights for questionnaires, of which the Rosser Index is perhaps the best known and the EuroQol is perhaps, at least within Europe, the most widely used measure.

The Rosser Index was gained from an initial survey of 60 doctors from a range of specialities which revealed that the primary criteria used to assess the severity of health states were disability and distress.[1] Disability referred to loss of physical and social functioning objectively assessed, whereas distress was classified by subjective evaluation of factors such as pain and psychological condition. Using the information gleaned from this survey and from subsequent discussions and testing with doctors, disability was ultimately classified into eight states, ranging from unconsciousness to no disability, and distress was classified into four groups, from severe to no distress. Figure 5.1 reports Rosser's categories.

Disability

1 No disability
2 Slight social disability
3 Severe social disability and/or slight impairment of performance at work. Able to do all housework except very heavy tasks
4 Choice of work or performance at work very severely limited. Housewives and old people able to do light housework only, but able to go out shopping
5 Unable to undertake any paid employment. Unable to continue any education. Old people confined to home except for escorted outings and short walks and unable to do shopping. Housewives only able to perform a few simple tasks
6 Confined to chair or to wheelchair or able to move around in the home only with support from an assistant
7 Confined to bed
8 Unconscious

Distress

A No distress
B Mild
C Moderate
D Severe

Figure 5.1 Rosser's classification of states of sickness.

These 12 states were combined to generate 29 health states. It was assumed that unconsciousness created no distress for the patient, thereby eliminating three cells from the matrix. Consequently, state 1A represents a condition of perfect health and no distress, whereas state 7C indicates a patient who is bedridden and in moderate distress. Seventy subjects drawn from six groups, including psychiatric and medical patients, experienced doctors, psychiatric and general nurses and 20 healthy volunteers, were then interviewed to elicit valuations for these 29 health states. Six states (1C, 2D, 5B, 6B, 7B and 7D) were selected as the 'marker states' to represent the full range of conditions. Subjects were initially asked to rank these six states in order of severity. They were told that the patients in these states were all the same age (e.g. young adults) and, in the first instance, that these people would be cured if they were treated but would remain in these states until another condition intervened if they were ignored. Subjects were then asked to assess the relative severity of successive pairs of marker states. The ratio 1:x between states was intended to reflect, first, the relative proportions of NHS resources which would be needed to equate the two states and, secondly, the point at which subjects were indifferent between curing one person in the more severe state and x people in the relatively healthier state.

Once the relationship between marker states had been established, respondents were then asked to evaluate the remaining 23 health states. At a later stage of interviews, the initial assumptions that these conditions could be cured were revised, but this produced little change in the relative values ascribed. Respondents were also asked to add a valuation for death.[2] Median values of the final scores were subsequently transformed so that a score of 0 was attributed to death and perfect health with no distress (state 1A) was scored at 1. These values have formed the basis for many QALY assessments even though the index was not originally designed with this purpose in mind. Two health states gained values less than 0 (i.e. confined to bed in severe distress, and unconscious). Negative values refer to conditions which are regarded as being worse than death.

Despite the wide application of the Rosser Index in QALY estimates, work has continued to revise these evaluations of life quality. In part this is due to the original valuations being based on such a small and potentially unrepresentative group of respondents. More recent developments have included, for example, work based on the original Rosser classifications of health states, but tested using different measures of utility assessment such as the time trade-off and standard gamble techniques outlined above.[3] Rosser also developed an instrument to measure health-related quality of life, the Index of Health-Related Quality of Life (IHQL), which is based on a multidimensional classification of health status developed from the original Rosser classification. In the new index, distress is subdivided into two categories of physical distress (discomfort) and emotional distress, allowing the description of 175 composite health states. These categories are subdivided further according to seven attributes and then by 44 scales. The IHQL explicitly aims to present a health state evaluation as a unified aggregate score but combine with it the advantages of clinical instruments providing profiles of subjective health assessment.[4] However, use of the Rosser Index and uptake of modified forms of the measure have been overshadowed in more recent years by the development and application of the EuroQol EQ-5D.

The EuroQol Group[5] was explicitly formed with the intention of developing a measure of health-related quality of life which could be expressed as a single value to facilitate cost-effectiveness analysis, but also retained the benefits of profile assessment. Researchers from a range of disciplines and European countries sought to construct an instrument which could be employed in parallel with the growing bank of tests already available, but which could act as a kind of 'gold standard' permitting the translation of individual scores on existing tests into an index which could be used for international comparisons. A further objective was to design a measure which could be applied relatively easily and presented so that subjects' responses would not be contaminated by fatigue or inadequate comprehension.[6]

The descriptive system which provided the framework for the EuroQol was derived from several existing instruments for health status measurement, including the Rosser Index (see above), the Nottingham Health Profile and Sickness Impact Profile (*see* Chapter 4) and the Quality of Well-Being Scale, the latter itself being a single-index measure of health status for use in health economic assessments of medical treatments but relatively complex to administer and score.[7] Ultimately five dimensions were defined, which were subdivided into three levels according to whether the dimension represented no problem, a moderate problem or a severe problem. The five dimensions were mobility, self-care, usual activity, pain and mood. The five-dimension, three-level classification system generated 243 (i.e. $3 \times 3 \times 3 \times 3 \times 3$) health states, which were extended to 245 with the addition of death and unconsciousness.

The valuation methodology that was initially adopted used a visual analogue scale, rather than the more complex time trade-off or standard gamble techniques. Subjects were asked to value 16 health states and to indicate on a 'thermometer' (which was graded from 'Worst Possible State' at 0 to 'Best Possible State' (perfect health) at 100) the value they assigned to the health state. Values were determined by drawing a line from the box describing the condition to the relevant point on the thermometer. However, the largest set of valuations was gained from a large-scale survey of the adult population of England, Scotland and Wales which adopted the time trade-off methodology.[8]

The instrument itself asked subjects to tick one of three boxes corresponding to each of the levels for the five dimensions. These could then be converted into a health state with an associated quality of life valuation. For example, the state 32312 would describe a patient who was confined to bed, experiencing some problems with washing and dressing, was unable to perform her usual activities, in no pain and suffering moderate depression. If this state were valued at, say, 65 then it would imply that the quality of a life in this condition should be weighted at 0.65 relative to a life in perfect health. Subjects completing the instrument (rather than the initial valuation surveys) were also asked to indicate on a scale what they considered their current health state to be. From this, some measure of the difference between individual perceptions of health status and socially determined valuations could be recognized. This would allow interventions to be evaluated on the basis of community preferences, which might be the most appropriate valuations for determining resource allocations, and individual preferences, which would allow the impact of interventions on the individuals concerned to be assessed.[6]

The considerable work that has gone into developing the EuroQol means that it has increasingly become one of the most widely adopted outcome measures in Europe. It has been found to be a practical and easy way of measuring health and capable of detecting, at least at the population level, differences in health in a meaningful manner.[9]

However, on the other hand, several problems have been raised in relation to the EuroQol measure. First, presentational problems have been identified which suggest that differences in the number of boxes representing the various conditions presented per page, and variations in the length of the thermometer, influence the valuations for some states. In addition, valuations proved to be vulnerable to the declared purpose for the scale: respondents tended to record higher scores for the more severe conditions if they were told that the index would be used to inform resource allocations than if they were simply told to consider the states as referring to 'people like you'.[6]

Some respondents also recorded inconsistent ratings. If states differed only to the extent that the level recorded for one dimension was lower in state B than state A, subjects should place B at a lower position on the thermometer than A. These inconsistencies were found to be particularly problematic when the only dimension to change was pain.[10] Inconsistent responses seemed most likely to occur with elderly or poorly educated respondents,[6] suggesting that the valuations might also be vulnerable to sample selection bias. In addition, these kinds of problems may suggest that the EuroQol has not achieved the level of crosscultural validity initially desired in the pursuit of an acceptable 'gold standard' measure which could be used for international comparisons.

Some evidence has also been forthcoming that the EuroQol is not sensitive to health changes that are of importance to patients.[11] However, more evidence is needed on this important issue from a wide variety of disease groups before the measure is dismissed.

At a more theoretical level, Carr-Hill has also criticized the use of composite health states, rather than a weighted average of scores for the individual dimensions.[12] He suggests that subjects are not likely to regard these components as being of equal significance in determining a health state, but it is difficult to disentangle these influences if valuations are based on composite conditions. Furthermore, the interpretation of some of the key states valued in the pilot surveys may be made more difficult if respondents try to relate them to real conditions. The difficulty in comprehending what these states mean may increase the variance in individual valuations.

EuroQol researchers have responded to these criticisms by reiterating the importance of their initial objectives and acknowledging that since their work is still in progress, many of these problems have yet to be addressed effectively. The instrument has not been developed to the point where health managers can adopt it uncritically,[5] but the importance of the questions raised by this project justifies the attempt to improve this index.

Many of the other criticisms levelled at the EuroQol focus more on the potential weaknesses of cost-utility analysis and the apparent assumption that preferences for given health states do not change over time. As Gafni and Birch remark, the assumptions of the cost-utility analysis and the QALY approach are analogous to assuming that the 100th hour of watching soccer on television is of the same value or 'utility' as watching the first hour, all other things being equal (one assumes that when they claim 'all other things being equal', they are referring to, for example, the quality of the play not changing over 100 hours).[13] There is precious little evidence to support assumptions such as these in relation to health state.

The difficulties posed by the problems of measuring utility in the EuroQol Project indicate such an undertaking is no easy task. However, the importance of the undertaking may be easy to dismiss but the real issue of limited resources and almost insatiable demand for health care means such approaches cannot be ignored forever. Attempts to measure health status in a manner that can be married up with costs may have so far proved unsatisfactory but the problem is unlikely to go away. Cost containment has always occurred in health care systems: health economics is at least trying to place the decisions on a more scientific basis.

Patient-generated measures

Consideration of outcome measures thus far has given examples of questionnaire which are based on fixed format questions with fixed format sets of responses. It has been suggested that such questionnaires may provide only a limited insight into the true quality of life of individuals experiencing health problems. Thus, while many of the instruments described in this text have been developed by assessing health-related aspects of quality of life in groups of individuals, the items selected for inclusion in the final questionnaires may not reflect the specific concerns of any one individual. It is difficult to determine what aspects of life are health related and what are not for different individuals. For instance, income or standard of living may be directly related to health in economies which have lower levels of social welfare to support people in ill health. They may also be more relevant to self-employed than to company-employed individuals in the same system. Furthermore, the weighting given to each item in scoring the questionnaires may not reflect the relative value of that aspect of health for a particular individual. For instance, ability to walk specific distances may have very different meanings for a sedentary television enthusiast and a hill-walking enthusiast. Yet their scores on standard questionnaires, e.g. if both report that they cannot walk more than a few streets as a result of their angina, would indicate an equivalent impact of illness on their health status. Because of these concerns, some researchers have attempted to develop instruments which are quantifiable but also individualized, i.e. they allow flexibility so that those aspects of life considered important by the individual being evaluated are included and the relative value of the different aspects selected is determined.[14] Two examples of these measures are described below: the Schedule for the Evaluation of Individual Quality of Life (SEIQoL)[15,16] and the Patient-Generated Index of Quality of Life (PGI).[17,18,19]

The SEIQoL is a semistructured interview and may be completed by both patients and the general population. It is completed in three stages. In the first stage, respondents are asked to list the five areas of life they judge to be most important in assessing overall quality of life. Those who find it difficult to list five areas are provided with a prompt list of eight possibilities (e.g. family, relationships). In the second stage, they rate their current status in each nominated area on a visual analogue scale from 'As good as could possibly be' to 'As bad as could possibly be'. The interviewer then generates a bar chart profile based on these assessments and asks the individual to rate their overall quality of life on a single visual analogue scale. In the third stage, respondents are presented with 30 hypothetical profiles randomly generated by computer. These are displayed as bar charts and labelled with the individual respondent's nominated areas. They are then asked to rate the overall quality of life score associated with each profile on a visual analogue scale. From these ratings, it is possible to estimate the relative weight attached to each nominated area using a statistical procedure called multiple regression analysis. Finally, an overall quality of life score for each individual is calculated by multiplying each nominated area by its corresponding weight and summing across the five areas to produce an index score between 0 and 100. A shorter method involves asking individuals to complete stages. The procedure can be time consuming and consequently a shorter method has also been developed.[20] This involves asking individuals to complete stages 1 and 2 as above and then presenting them with a disk comprising five stacked, centrally mounted interlocking laminated disks, each a different colour and labelled to represent one of the nominated life areas. The disks can be rotated over each other to produce a dynamic pie chart. Respondents rotate the overlapping disks until they are satisfied that they represent the relative weights they assign to the different areas they have nominated.[20] The relative weight can then be read from a 0–100-point scale on the outer rim of the disk. These values are used for weighting in the calculation of the overall index score. However, this shorter form version has to date been used relatively infrequently.

The PGI was developed for use in routine clinical practice and was therefore designed as a self-completed questionnaire. Because of the nature of its design, the PGI cannot be administered to healthy people and therefore cannot be used to generate comparative norms. Like the SEIQoL, the PGI is completed in three stages. The first stage asks patients to list the five most important areas or activities of their life affected by their condition. The second stage asks patients to rate how badly affected they are in each of their chosen areas on a scale of 0 to 100, where 0 represents the worst they can imagine for themselves and 100 represents exactly as they would like to be. A sixth box is provided to enable them to rate all other areas of their life not previously mentioned. This may include areas of their life affected by their medical condition but not important enough to be included in the top five boxes as well as areas which might be unrelated to their condition or even to their health. In the third stage, they are asked to imagine that they can improve some or all of the chosen areas of their life. They are 'given' 60 'points' which they can choose to spend across one or more areas, reflecting the relative importance they attach to potential improvements in those areas. Finally, by multiplying each of the six ratings by the proportion of points allocated to that area and summing, an index is generated between 0 and 100.

A comparison of the SEIQoL and PGI

The SEIQoL and the PGI are conceptually quite similar. They both allow patients to define quality of life in a way that has meaning for them, to assess the extent to which reality departs from their own expectations and to value the relative importance of improvement in their chosen areas of life. However, there are important differences between the two methods. The SEIQoL asks patients to nominate the five most important areas of life, while the PGI asks for the most important areas of life affected by the medical condition and two different techniques are used to elicit the relative weights for the chosen areas. Before an instrument can be recommended for use as an evaluative quality of life measure, empirical evidence is required to establish its validity, reliability, responsiveness to change and practicability as a routine tool in quality of life assessment.

The test-retest reliability of the SEIQoL has been assessed in a sample of 20 control subjects selected from a general practitioner list, as part of a prospective study of unilateral total hip replacement.[15] These controls were matched for age, sex and socioeconomic status with 20 patients undergoing surgery. They completed the SEIQoL in their homes on two occasions 32 weeks apart. On the second occasion, subjects were provided with their original five chosen areas and asked to generate new ratings and weights. The test-retest reliability coefficient indicated a high level of reliability.

PGI test-retest reliability has been assessed in a sample of 111 patients experiencing low back pain.[17] A postal version of the PGI was mailed to patients on two occasions separated by a two-week interval. The second questionnaire included a question asking patients if their health had improved, got worse or remained the same since completing the first questionnaire. For patients reporting no change in health between the first and second set of responses, a good test-retest reliability coefficient was gained, although not quite as high as that found for the SEIQoL.

Both the SEIQoL and the PGI exceed the level of test-retest reliability which has been cited as required for group comparisons.[21] Indeed, the very high reliability coefficient obtained for the SEIQoL suggests that it may also be suitable for monitoring quality of life in individuals.[22] This result is particularly impressive when one considers the 32-week interval between administrations. However, in the SEIQoL study, subjects were provided with their previous chosen areas when completing their second interview while in the PGI study, patients completed the retest questionnaire without recourse to their initial responses (with the result that patients made an average 1.7 changes in their choice of areas).[17] It is possible that a higher reliability coefficient could be obtained for the PGI if, as in the SEIQoL study, patients were provided with their previous responses when completing follow-up questionnaires. It has been suggested that this approach leads to an artificial improvement in reliability, with respondents repeating their previous response irrespective of any true change.[23] If this were so, any improvement in reliability would be accompanied by a reduction in responsiveness to change. However, Guyatt found this not to be the case in his study of patients with chronic cardiorespiratory disease.[24]

The criterion validity of the SEIQoL and PGI has been assessed. In the SEIQoL hip replacement study,[15] patients' health status was assessed using a general measure of health – the generic McMaster Health Index Questionnaire (MHIQ)[25] – and a condition-specific measure of disease – the Arthritis Impact Measurement Scale (AIMS).[26] Whilst correlations were found between the SEIQoL and these other, standardized measures, they were low, which has been interpreted as indicating that the SEIQoL is measuring aspects of the same phenomenon as measured on the MHIQ and AIMS, but is not measuring exactly the same thing. A similar approach was taken for the PGI. In the PGI study of low back pain, health status was also assessed with a combination of general and disease-specific measures. General health was measured by the Short Form 36-item Health Survey Questionnaire (see Chapter 4) and the severity of low back pain was assessed by the Aberdeen Low Back Pain Scale[27] which is a 19-item questionnaire devised from questions commonly used in the clinical assessment of patients presenting with low back pain. Patients' scores on the PGI demonstrated significant correlations with all eight SF-36 scales but were not correlated very highly. For both the SEIQoL and PGI, the degree of correlation with established health status measures reported in these studies lends support to claims made by the instruments' authors that they assess quality of life. However, a more critical interpretation might be that seeking 'some form of correlation' is not a very hard test to pass. Indeed, some of the significance levels chosen as acceptable were very low and one might be surprised if measures hadn't passed these tests!

Perhaps more convincing data come in the form of tests for construct validity. The developers of the SEIQoL have assessed construct validity by focusing on the various methods employed to derive a SEIQoL quality of life score, rather than testing the validity of the final score itself.[15] From data provided by the SEIQoL hip replacement study, for example, the following hypotheses were tested: SEIQoL scores using pre-determined areas or activities of life derived from traditional health status measures are less sensitive to improvement in quality of life following surgery compared with SEIQoL scores using areas elicited by patients; individuals vary considerably in the relative importance they attach to the five areas as reflected in the weights they assign to each; and for a given individual the relative importance of each area may change over time.

Although the most frequently mentioned areas – such as, for example, social/leisure activities, family and personal health – will be found in most conventional health status questionnaires, certain areas elicited by the SEIQoL, e.g. religion, finances, family health, would not normally be included. When patients undergoing hip replacement completed the SEIQoL using five pre-determined areas of life – physical functioning, social functioning, emotional functioning, living conditions and general health – derived from conventional questionnaires, a non-significant improvement in quality of life score was detected seven and a half months after surgery.[15] When SEIQoL scores were generated using patients' own elicited areas of life, a statistically significant improvement was detected.[15] Considerable variation was found between individuals in the weights assigned to different areas of life when respondents were asked to complete the SEIQoL using the five pre-determined areas.[15] There was also evidence that patients changed the relative importance attached to certain areas over time.

If a quality of life measure is to be used to evaluate the outcome of care for patients, then it must be shown to be responsive, or sensitive, to clinically significant change in quality of life over time (*see* Chapter 3). In the SEIQoL hip replacement study, quality of life was measured in 20 patients during routine pre-surgical assessment six weeks prior to surgery and again 26 weeks post-operatively. In the PGI low back pain study, 136 patients were assessed within two weeks of consulting their general practitioner and again after one year. Responsiveness, measured using the effect size statistic, showed moderate to substantial change. In another study of treatment for sleep apnoea,[28] PGI scores were compared to scores on standardized measures. The PGI indicated substantial change whereas standardized measures did not. This could be explained by the fact that patients nominate areas they believe are the most appropriate for themselves and which may not be assessed on conventional fixed-item questionnaires. However, it could also be argued that individualized measures are overly sensitive to small but effectively fairly unimportant changes.

An instrument intended for use as an outcome measure should not only satisfy psychometric criteria of validity, reliability and responsiveness as discussed above; practical considerations are also important. The range of populations which can be assessed, the time taken to complete and score instruments and the need for personnel to assist with assessment are all important considerations. The SEIQoL is applicable in most clinical situations with adults and completion rates have been found to be very high, with in some cases 100% completion. Furthermore, because it can be administered to healthy individuals, normative values can be derived for comparative purposes. However, it is interviewer administered and the original version takes about 30 minutes to complete while the shorter form direct weighting procedure takes about 15 minutes. This limits the use of these outcome measures in busy clinical settings. The PGI can also be administered by an interviewer with almost 100% completion rates. The major practical advantage of the PGI over the SEIQoL, however, is in its use as a self-administered postal questionnaire but use of the postal PGI has been associated with somewhat low response rates. Another potential limitation with the PGI is that normative values cannot be derived for the PGI as the measure is designed to assess the impact of ill health on quality of life; consequently, one cannot complete it if one is in good health.

The opportunity for respondents to select their own areas of health status for inclusion in a questionnaire is an exciting and potentially valuable development. However, the questionnaires can be difficult to complete and ideally require someone to help administer them, whereas standard form measures simply require respondents to tick boxes. Furthermore, there exists an assumption that analysing these data at a group level is acceptable despite the fact that different respondents select different items to include in their own individualized measures. The fact that one might be adding up apples and oranges (i.e. unrelated phenomena) rather than aspects of a single unitary concept of 'quality of life' must at least be a possibility. However, there is nonetheless something intuitively appealing about this approach.

Summary

Index measures of outcomes provide a single number which supposedly reflects the health status of an individual. However, as this chapter has shown, very different approaches to gaining such a single number have evolved. Some developers favour measures based upon societal values, whilst others feel that quality of life is such an individual phenomenon that it should be measured explicitly at the level of the individual. The applications of the two methodologies are radically different. More research is needed from both sides to gain a full appreciation of the pros and cons of these approaches. At the present time users must decide carefully which approach is the most appropriate. For example, in a trial of two competing but identically priced drugs the PGI may be an appropriate measure but in a cost-utility analysis, the EuroQol would be more suitable. However, before either methodology is used uncritically, more information on the operating characteristics of these measures seems to be required.

References

1 Rosser R (1988) A health index and output measure. In: *Quality of Life: assessment and application* (eds SR Walker, RM Rosser), MTP Press, Lancaster.

2 Rosser R, Kind P (1978) A scale of valuations of states of illness. Is there a social consensus? *International Journal of Epidemiology.* 7: 247–58.

3 Gudex C, Kind P, van Dalen H *et al.* (1993) *Comparing Scaling Methods for Health State Valuations – Rosser revisited.* Working paper no. 107. Centre for Health Economics, University of York.

4 Rosser R, Cottee M, Rabin R, Selai C (1992) Index of health-related quality of life. In: *Measures of the Quality of Life and the Uses to Which Such Measures May be Put* (ed A Hopkins), Royal College of Physicians of London, London.

5 EuroQol Group (1990) EuroQol – a new facility for the measurement of health-related quality of life. *Health Policy.* 16: 199–208.

6 Kind P (1996) The EuroQol instrument: an index of health-related quality of life. In: *Quality of Life and Pharmacoeconomics in Clinical Trials,* 2nd edn (ed B Spilker), Lippincott-Raven, Philadelphia.

7 Kaplan R, Anderson JP, Ganiats G (1993) The Quality of Well-Being Scale: rationale for a single quality of life index. In: *Quality of Life Assessment: key issues in the 1990s* (eds S Walker, R Rosser), Kluwer, London.

8 Williams A (1995) *The Measurement and Valuation of Health: a Chronicle.* Discussion Paper 136. Centre for Health Economics, University of York.

9   Kind P, Dolan P, Gudex C, Williams A (1998) Variations in populations health status: results from a United Kingdom national questionnaire survey. *British Medical Journal.* **316**: 736–41.
10 Carr-Hill R (1992) A second opinion. Health related quality of life – Euro style. *Health Policy.* **16**: 321–8.
11 Jenkinson C, Gray A, Doll H *et al.* (1997) Evaluation of index and profile measures of health status in a randomised controlled trial: comparison of the SF-36, EuroQol and disease specific measures. *Medical Care.* **35**: 1109–18.
12 Carr-Hill R (1992) A second opinion. Health related quality of life measurement – Euro style. *Health Policy.* **20**: 321–8.
13 Gafni A, Birch S (1993) Searching for a common currency: critical appraisal of the scientific basis underlying European harmonisation of health related quality of life (EuroQol). *Health Policy.* **23**: 219–28.
14 Joyce CRB, O'Boyle CA, McGee HM (eds) (1998) *Individual Quality of Life Assessment in Health Care.* Harwood Academic, Reading.
15 O'Boyle CA, McGee H, Hickey A, O'Malley K, Joyce CRB (1992) Individual quality of life in patients undergoing hip replacement. *Lancet.* **339**: 1088–91.
16 McGee H, O'Boyle CA, Hickey A, O'Malley K, Joyce CRB (1991) Assessment of quality of life in the individual: the SEIQoL with a healthy and gastroenterology unit population. *Psychological Medicine.* **21**: 749–59.
17 Ruta D, Garratt AM, Leng M, Russell IT, Macdonald LM (1994) A new approach to the measurement of quality of life: the Patient Generated Index (PGI). *Medical Care.* **32**: 1109–23.
18 Ruta D, Garratt A (1994) Health status to quality of life measurement. In: *Measuring Health and Medical Outcomes* (ed C Jenkinson), UCL Press, London.
19 Garratt A, Ruta D (1996) Taking a patient centred approach to outcome measurement. In: *Health Outcome Measures in Primary and Out-Patient Care* (eds A Hutchinson, E McColl, M Christie, C Riccalton), Harwood Academic, Amsterdam.
20 Hickey A, Bury G, O'Boyle CA *et al.* (1996) A new short-form individual quality of life measure (SEIQoL-DW): application in a cohort of individuals with HIV/AIDS. *British Medical Journal.* **313**: 29–33.
21 Streiner DL, Norman GR (1995) *Health Measurement Scales: a guide to their development and use,* 2nd edn. Oxford University Press, Oxford.
22 Kelly TL (1927) *Interpretation of Educational Measurements.* World Book Publishing, New York.

23 Jacobsen M (1965) The use of rating scales in clinical research. *British Journal of Psychiatry.* **111**: 545–6.
24 Guyatt G, Berman LB, Townsend M, Taylor DW (1985) Should study subjects see their previous responses? *Journal of Chronic Diseases.* **38**: 1003–7.
25 Chambers L (1993) The McMaster Health Index Questionnaire: an update. In: *Quality of Life Assessment: key issues in the 1990s* (eds SR Walker, R Rosser), Kluwer, London.
26 Meenan RF (1982) The AIMS approach to health status measurement: conceptual background and measurement properties. *Journal of Rheumatology.* **9**: 785–8.
27 Ruta D, Garratt A, Wardlow I, Russell IT (1994) Developing a valid and reliable measure of health outcome for patients with low back pain. *Spine.* **19**: 1887–96.
28 Jenkinson C, Stradling J, Petersen S (1998) How should we evaluate health status? A comparison of three methods in patients presenting with obstructive sleep apnoea. *Quality of Life Research.* **7**: 95–100.

6
Disease-specific measures

Introduction

Disease-specific measures are questionnaires designed specifically to target a particular patient group. They may provide a profile of scores, such as in the Kidney Disease Questionnaire,[1] an index, such as the Oxford Hip Score,[2] or both, as in the case of the Parkinson's Disease Questionnaire.[3] Profile measures provide a number of scores across a wide variety of areas that the illness may affect, whilst index measures summarize data into a single figure.

Disease-specific measures exist for a wide variety of conditions and health states. The advantage of disease-specific measures of outcome over generic health status measures is that, ideally, they should measure aspects of ill health that are particularly salient to the disease group being studied and they should therefore be more sensitive to changes. This has been supported in a number of studies where, for example, generic measures have failed to indicate change as a consequence of treatment but disease-specific measures have done so.[4] The purpose of this chapter is to outline the most commonly adopted developmental procedures which can be used to produce a disease-specific measure.

Developing disease-specific measures

Guyatt and colleagues have suggested two broad approaches to the development and testing of disease-specific measures.[5] Table 6.1 outlines the broad principles that could be used to develop a so called 'Rolls-Royce' disease-specific measure or a simpler 'Volkswagen' model for use in clinical trials. Whilst the procedures recommended are for disease-specific measures for use primarily in trials, the design principles seem appropriate for the development of any disease-specific measure irrespective of its intended applications.

Broadly speaking, items must first be generated for a questionnaire. This will ideally involve semistructured interviews with patients who will provide information on the impact of the illness on their lives. However, many disease specific questionnaires have been based upon reviews of the literature, although this is not always satisfactory as much literature on patients' quality of life is based upon clinical assessment. When in-depth interviews with patients are undertaken the statements to be used in the questionnaire will be based upon patient report, which must be viewed as the 'gold standard' for gaining information on the experience of almost any illness. Reduction of the amount of items generated from such numbers can be undertaken in a number of ways. Guyatt and colleagues suggest finding the items most frequently cited as well as those nominated by patients as the most important. On the other hand, statistical procedures can be employed to reduce the number of items. This will be discussed below. The questionnaire must then undergo preliminary testing for acceptability to patients and then the validity, reliability and sensitivity to change must be assessed. It is possible to forego the latter stages but increasingly questionnaires which do so are not seen as acceptable and consequently alternatives are sought.

To highlight the practicalities of developing a questionnaire following a 'Rolls Royce' model, we outline below the development of the Parkinson's Disease Questionnaire designed primarily to assess outcomes in trials of therapies for Parkinson's disease (PD). Other procedures exist but this is perhaps the most commonly used.

Development of a questionnaire – an example

Parkinson's disease is a common neurological condition which can have substantial implications for the health and well-being of patients. However, traditionally the progress of the disease has been monitored using scales completed by clinicians. This overlooks the patient's perspective and consequently must be seen, in the context of evaluating treatments, as a limited form of assessment. The Parkinson's Disease Questionnaire was developed as a disease-specific measure for use primarily in clinical trials. The development and validation processes are outlined below.

To ensure that the questionnaire captured aspects of health status important to patients, in-depth interviews were conducted with 20

Stage	Rolls-Royce model	Volkswagen model
Item selection	Literature review Comprehensive consultation with health professionals Use of existing measures Interviews with 50–100 patients	Use of existing measures Consultation with health professionals
Reduction of no. of items	Choose items most frequently mentioned by patients Use of statisticsl techniques (e.g. factor analysis to select items)	Include the items gained in item selection
Questionnaire format	Select response options Specify time range	Select response options Specify time range
Pre-test	Pre-test on 20 or more patients	Pre-test on 2 or 3 patients
Sampling for the above procedures	Use representative sample covering as wide a range of patient attributes as possible	Use a convenience sample
Test-retest	Administer questionnaire twice to stable patients	None
Sensitivity to change	Administer before and after a treatment of known efficacy	None
Validity	Check for construct validity (see Chapter 3) based on a priori predictions	Use face validity (i.e. does the measure appear to make sense?)

Table 6.1 Stages in the development of two models for measuring quality of life (adapted from Guyatt et al.[5]).

people with PD attending a neurology outpatient clinic. People were asked to describe the areas of their lives which had been adversely affected by their PD. This generated a large number of possible questionnaire items which could be included in the final questionnaire. These items were scrutinized for ambiguity and repetition. A 65-item questionnaire was developed and piloted to test basic acceptability and comprehension.

The next stage was to reduce the number of questionnaire items and generate scales for the different dimensions of health-related quality of life. Three hundred and fifty nine individuals completed the 65-item questionnaire, from which factor analyses produced a 39-item questionnaire with eight dimensions. Reliability in terms of internal consistency of each dimension was assessed using the Cronbach's alpha statistic (see Chapter 3). Internal consistency was found to be good for all dimensions. The result was the PDQ-39, a questionnaire with 39 items

---

Dimensions

Mobility
Activities of daily living
Emotional well-being
Stigma
Social support
Cognitions
Communication

An overall score can also be calculated

Table 6.2 Dimensions on the Parkinson's
Disease Questionnaire.

covering eight dimensions (Table 6.2). The scores from each dimension are computed into a scale ranging from 0 (Best, i.e. no problem at all) through to 100 (Worst, i.e. maximum level of problem).

The measurement properties of the PDQ-39, in terms of reliability, validity and sensitivity to change, were assessed by using data from a second postal survey and an outpatient clinic sample. For the second postal survey, all members with PD from five different PDS branches were posted a booklet containing the PDQ-39, the SF-36, and questions about the severity of their PD symptoms. In addition, a second copy of the PDQ-39 was included in a sealed envelope. Respondents were asked to complete the second copy 3–6 days after the first and to report any important changes in their health during that time. In the clinic sample, individuals with PD attending as neurology outpatients were surveyed with the PDQ-39 and the SF-36 and clinically assessed using the Hoehn and Yahr Index[6] and the Columbia Rating Scale,[7] which are both established clinical measures of outcome in PD, and were reassessed with the same measures four months later.

The reliability of the PDQ was assessed using Cronbach's alpha statistic and test-retest reliability (see Chapter 3 for more information on these tests). The two sets of PDQ-39 data from the second postal survey were obtained in order to examine reliability in terms of internal consistency of the eight PDQ-39 dimensions. Cronbach's alpha was satisfactory for all scales on both occasions. Test-retest reliability (reproducibility) was examined by means of correlation coefficients between scale scores at time 1 and time 2. The data were highly correlated and not statistically different, indicating good levels of reliability.

Construct validity was examined by means of correlations of scale scores with relevant SF-36 scores. Significant correlations were found between matching scales of the PDQ-39 and the SF-36. Questionnaire items asked respondents to assess severity of their tremor, stiffness and slowness. A consistent pattern of worse scores on all PDQ-39 scales was obtained from patients with more severe self-assessed symptoms.

Validity of the PDQ-39 was also examined in terms of agreement with clinical assessments performed by the neurologists in the clinic study: the Hoehn and Yahr Index and the Columbia Rating Scale. Significant correlations were found between both clinical scales and the PDQ-39 dimensions for all dimensions except social support.

The sensitivity to change of a quality of life instrument is particularly important in view of potential applications in clinical trials. This was tested on data from the clinic sample in terms of whether changes in PDQ-39 scores over a four-month period were consistent with patients' global retrospective judgements of change. Change scores for the PDQ-39 were calculated as standardized response means (the change score for a measure divided by the standard deviation of that change score). Changes for two dimensions of the PDQ-39, mobility and ADL, were statistically significantly different and standardized response means (*see* Chapter 3) suggested moderate deterioration for the sample who described themselves as worse in their global retrospective judgements after four months. This suggests reasonable sensitivity to change for these two dimensions. For all patients, their retrospective judgement of change significantly correlated with change scores for mobility and ADL. More work on the sensitivity to change needs to be undertaken, although the slow progress of the disease means such studies tend to be very long term.

Subsequent analysis of the data has indicated that a single figure can also be gained from the PDQ-39. Those interested in this particular questionnaire are referred to specific publications on the development and validation of the measure.[3,8,9]

Summary

The development of a disease-specific questionnaire with rigorous measurement properties is a fairly time-consuming business. However, the resulting measure should truly tap aspects of particular interest to the patient group under study and should be sensitive to changes in health which are of particular concern to them. Nonetheless, interpretation is often difficult as it is not possible to 'norm' against a general population sample. Many instruments have been compared to clinical measures and the scores can be interpreted in the light of such comparison. This enables clinicians to gain some insight as to what the data from the measures mean, but this can lead to health status profiles being standardized against clinical rating scales, which somewhat defeats the object of creating patient-based measures. Furthermore, patient report and clinical judgement are sometimes at odds with one another. Another possible way to gain insight into the meanings of scores is to simply see what items need to be affirmed (or not) to lead to certain sets of scores. This is known as content-based interpretation. Ways of assessing the sensitivity and meaningfulness of scores are discussed in depth in Chapter 3.

It should be stressed that disease-specific measures are not intended to replace generic measures but to complement them. Thus data can be gained on aspects of specific importance to specific patient groups as well as data on how they score in relation to the general population on a generic measure. Use of disease-specific measures alone does not permit such comparisons and, furthermore, even when they can be summed to a single index they cannot be used in cost-utility studies (because, by definition, data from disease-specific measures cannot be compared with other patient groups).

Finally users should carefully consider which disease-specific measure to employ. There are many diseases where more than one measure exists and informed choices should be made. Chapter 7 suggests some criteria that must be assessed when selecting between competing instruments. Reference books are available that provide information on many of the different scales applicable to a wide variety of conditions,[10–14] as are regularly updated computer databases.[15, 16]

References

1 Laupacis A, Muirhead N, Keown P, Wong C (1992) A disease specific questionnaire for assessing quality of life in patients on haemodialysis. *Nephron.* **60**: 302–6.

2 Dawson J, Fitzpatrick R, Carr A, Murray A (1996) Questionnaire on the perceptions of patients about total hip replacement therapy. *Journal of Bone and Joint Surgery.* **78B**: 185–90.

3 Jenkinson C, Fitzpatrick R, Peto V (1998) *The Parkinson's Disease Questionnaire: user manual for the PDQ-39, PDQ-8 and PDQ Summary Index.* Health Services Research Unit, Oxford.

4 Jenkinson C, Gray A, Doll H *et al.* (1997) Evaluation of index and profile measures of health status in a randomised controlled trial:

comparison of the SF-36, EuroQol and disease specific measures. *Medical Care*. **35**: 1109–18.

5   Guyatt GH, Bombardier C, Tugwell PX (1986) Measuring disease-specific quality of life in clinical trials. *Canadian Medical Association Journal*. **134**: 889–95.

6   Hoehn MM, Yahr MD (1967) Parkinsonism: onset, progression and mortality. *Neurology*. **17**: 427–42.

7   Hely MA, Chey T, Wilson A *et al.* (1993) Reliability of the Columbia Scale for assessing signs of Parkinson's disease. *Movement Disorders*. **8**: 466–72.

8   Peto V, Jenkinson C, Fitzpatrick R, Greenhall, R (1995) The development and validation of a short measure of functioning and well-being for individuals with Parkinson's disease. *Quality of Life Research*. **4**: 241–8.

9   Jenkinson C, Peto V, Fitzpatrick R, Greenhall R, Hyman, N (1995) Self reported functioning and well being in patients with Parkinson's disease: comparison of the Short Form Health Survey (SF-36) and the Parkinson's Disease Questionnaire (PDQ-39). *Age and Ageing*. **24**: 505–9.

10   Bowling A (1997) *Measuring Health: a review of quality of life measurement scales*, 2nd edn. Open University Press, Buckingham.

11   Bowling A (1995) *Measuring Disease*. Open University Press, Buckingham.

12   McDowell I, Newell C (1996) *Measuring Health: a guide to rating scales and questionnaires*, 2nd edn. Oxford University Press, New York.

13   Wilkin D, Hallam L, Doggett M (1992) *Measures of Need and Outcome for Primary Health Care*. Oxford University Press, Oxford.

14   Spilker B (1997) *Quality of Life and Pharmacoeconomics in Clinical Trials*, 2nd edn. Lippincott-Raven, Philadelphia.

15   Tamburini M. Quality of Life Assessment in Medicine: Bibliographic Reference. This CD disk is updated regularly and is available from Glamm Interactive Srl, Viale Corsica 7, 20133 Milan, Italy (e-mail qlam@glamm.com).

16   Staquet M. Quality of Life Updated Bibliography. This 3.5 inch disk is updated regularly and is available from M Staquet, Faculty of Medicine (DCS), CP623, Route de Lennik 8808, B-1070, Brussels, Belgium.

7
Conclusions: criteria for selecting measures

Introduction

The presentation of health status data in a published paper can often look scientific and rigorous in large part because it is presented in tabular form and analysed statistically. However, as the preceding chapters have suggested, such presentation can sometimes hide limitations with measures and inappropriate analysis. Consequently, researchers should select measures with care and explain why they have selected them and readers should look for evidence that some thought has been given to the inclusion of the measures used. In this final chapter we provide a brief guide to some of the issues that need to be considered when selecting a questionnaire or when reading a paper which includes data gained from a patient-based health outcome measure.

Criteria for selecting measures

A number of attempts have been made to suggest checklists of criteria to be used when selecting or appraising the quality of health status measures.[1,2] Tables 7.1 and 7.2 summarize some competing perspectives, although they reflect rather divergent and somewhat idiosyncratic attributes. For example, Gill and Feinstein's[1] criteria seem to assume that individualized measures are used (i.e. measures such as the SEIQoL and PGI discussed in Chapter 5), whilst Guyatt and Cook's[2] criteria overlook issues of acceptability and administration. Unfortunately, to date, no formal grading scheme has been developed which takes account of the competing views and perspectives of the wide variety of researchers in the field, although Fitzpatrick et al.[3] have, on the basis of a

Is quality of life conceptually defined?
Are domains to be measured explicitly stated?
Are selected outcome measures explained or justified?
Are scores aggregated into a single score?
Are patients able to offer a separate global score?
Is a distinction made between overall quality of life versus health-related quality of life?

Table 7.1 Requirements for judging the appropriateness of outcome measures I (adapted from Gill and Feinstein[1]).

Do the authors show that aspects of patients' lives measured are important to patients?
Have previous studies demonstrated their importance?
Do investigators examine aspects of patients' lives that, from clinical experience, it is known that patients value?
Have any aspects of health-related quality of life that are important to patients been omitted?
Are individual patients asked to place a value on their lives?
Have the instruments used been demonstrated to have reliability, validity and responsiveness?
Do instruments have interpretability?

Table 7.2 Requirements for judging the appropriateness of outcome measures II (adapted from Guyatt and Cook[2]).

systematic review, suggested eight questions that could reasonably form the basis of such a schema. These authors suggest that measures should be appropriate, reliable, valid, responsive, precise, interpretable, acceptable to patients and 'feasible'. Table 7.3 documents the eight questions that they suggest should be posed when selecting measures for inclusion in trials and although different criteria may need to be developed for assessing measures for use in other research designs, it is likely they will share similar attributes. A similar group of criteria were developed on the basis of a relatively small scale consultation exercise in the USA although they gave greater emphasis to the importance for good-quality translations, which retain the meaning of the questions, to exist or be undertaken when trials using such measures are international in nature.[4] However, this is effectively covered under 'acceptability' in Fitzpatrick *et al.*'s schema.

In summary, the following would seem to be the minimum criteria to be considered when assessing a questionnaire for inclusion in any study.

- Do the authors provide any evidence for the selection and inclusion of the measures in their study? For example, do they suggest why the instruments chosen are particularly appropriate, e.g. because normative data are available which may enable comparison with other populations and samples; because the questionnaire was designed for use in the particular group under study; because the instrument has been successfully used in the particular group under study in previous publications, etc.?

- Do the instruments included have proven reliability and validity? If so, is there any evidence that they are appropriate for use in the particular group under investigation?

- Is there any evidence that the measures will be sensitive to clinically or subjectively important changes? Related to this, what is the evidence, if any, for the precision of the instrument (i.e. ability to differentiate important differences in health state)?

- Are the questionnaires acceptable to patients (i.e. easy to understand and complete, not overly long or repetitive)?

Is the content of the measure **appropriate** to the questions which the clinical trial is intended to address?

Does the instrument produce **reliable** results (i.e. that are reproducible and internally consistent)?

Is the measure **valid** (i.e. does it measure what it claims to measure)?

Is the measure **responsive** (i.e. does the measure detect changes over time that matter to patients)?

How **precise** are the scores on the measure (i.e. how able is the measure to detect differences in health)?

How **interpretable** are the scores on the measure?

Is the measure **acceptable** to patients (e.g. is it too long or potentially distressing)?

How **feasible** is the measure for the study (i.e. is the instrument easy to administer and process)?

Table 7.3 Requirements for judging the appropriateness of outcome measures in clinical trials (adapted from Fitzpatrick et al.[3]).

Papers that do not attempt to address these issues must be regarded as potentially, although not necessarily, flawed. If health status measurement is to gain an ever-increasing role in health care evaluation it must, of course, be scientifically rigorous. This is not only true for the assessment of measures and research in which they are used, but also for papers documenting their development. These must also conform to certain minimum standards.[5] The purpose and conceptual basis of measures must be explicit, as must the manner in which they were constructed. If a measure is intended to quantify patient-based quality of life then it is important that questions included in the final instrument are, at least in part, derived from patients. The measure must be assessed for reliability, validity and sensitivity to change and, ideally, the developers should provide some indication as to how scores can be interpreted. Finally, the adoption and understanding of a measure is facilitated by the publishing of a user manual, which is relatively rare in this field.

Conclusions

This book has outlined the applications and potential limitations of health outcome measures. The potential for transforming assessment of health care and the practice of medicine will only be realized if people are thoughtful and critical in their choice of instruments and interpretation of results. Simply incorporating outcome measures into studies does not mean that the data will be meaningful or interesting. At present there is something of a tendency to include such measures rather uncritically, largely, it seems, because it is in vogue and seems to gain support from funding agencies. A more critical awareness of the issues in health status measurement will mean that uptake will increase and the fruits of the endeavour will be results that could have major and lasting impacts upon health care and medicine. The onus is on researchers to select questionnaires critically and, wherever possible, to minimize respondent burden by keeping them as brief as possible.

References

1 Gill TM, Feinstein AR (1994) A critical appraisal of the quality of quality of life instruments. *Journal of the American Medical Association.* **272**: 619–26.
2 Guyatt G, Cook DJ (1994) Health status, quality of life and the individual. *Journal of the American Medical Association.* **272**: 630–1.
3 Fitzpatrick R, Davey C, Buxton M, Jones D (1997) Evaluating Patient Based Outcome Measures for Use in Clinical Trials. Report submitted to the NHS Health Technology Assessment Programme.

4 Medical Outcomes Trust Scientific Advisory Committee (1995) Instrument review criteria. *Medical Outcomes Trust Bulletin.* **3** (4): I–IV.
5 McDowell I, Jenkinson C (1996) Development standards for health measures. *Journal of Health Services Research and Policy.* **1**: 238–46.

Recommended reading

For those who would like more information on the topics discussed in this book, the following texts are a good place to start.

General methodology

Bowling A (1997) *Research Methods in Health*. Open University Press, Buckingham.
Jenkinson C (ed) (1997) *Assessment and Evaluation of Health and Medical Care*. Open University Press, Buckingham.

Evidence-based medicine

Gray JAM (1997) *Evidence-Based Healthcare. How to Make Health Policy and Management Decisions*. Churchill Livingstone, London.
Lockett T (1997) *Evidence-Based and Cost-Effective Medicine for the Uninitiated*. Radcliffe Medical Press, Oxford.
Sackett DL, Richardson WS, Rosenberg W, Haynes RB (1997) *Evidence-Based Medicine. How to Practice and Teach EBM*. Churchill Livingstone, London.

Health economics

Brookes R (1995) *Health Status Measurement: a perspective on change*. Macmillan, London.
Lockett T (1996) *Health Economics for the Uninitiated*. Radcliffe Medical Press, Oxford.
Mooney G (1994) *Key Issues in Health Economics*. Harvester Wheatsheaf, Hemel Hempstead.

Questionnaire design

Oppenheim B (1992) *Questionnaire Design, Interviewing and Attitude Measurement*. Pinter, London.
Streiner DL, Norman GR (1995) *Health Measurement Scales: a practical guide to their development and use*, 2nd edn. Oxford University Press, Oxford.

Health status measurement – methodological considerations

Jenkinson C (ed) (1994) *Measuring Health and Medical Outcomes*. UCL Press, London.
O'Boyle CA, McGee H, Joyce CRB (1998) *Individual Quality of Life: approaches to conceptualisation and measurement in health*. Harwood, Reading.
Spilker B (ed) (1996) *Quality of Life and Pharmacoeconomics in Clinical Trials*, 2nd edn. Lippincott-Raven, Philadelphia.
Staquet M, Hays R, Fayers P (1998) *Quality of Life Assessment in Clinical Trials*. Oxford University Press, Oxford.
Streiner DL, Norman GR (1995) *Health Measurement Scales: a practical guide to their development and use*, 2nd edn. Oxford University Press, Oxford.

Health status measurement – applications

Albrecht GL, Fitzpatrick R (eds) (1994) *Quality of Life in Health Care. Advances in Medical Sociology, Volume 5*. JAI Press, Greenwich, Connecticut.
Fallowfield L (1990) *The Quality of Life*. Souvenir Press, London.
Spilker B (ed) (1996) *Quality of Life and Pharmacoeconomics in Clinical Trials*, 2nd edn. Lippincott-Raven, Philadelphia.

Health status measurement – compendiums and guides

Bowling A (1997) *Measuring Health: a review of quality of life measurement scales*, 2nd edn. Open University Press, Buckingham.
Bowling A (1995) *Measuring Disease: a review of disease specific quality of life scales*. Open University Press, Buckingham.
McDowell I, Newell C (1996) *Measuring Health: a guide to rating scales and questionnaires*, 2nd edn. Oxford University Press, Oxford.
Wilkin D, Hallam L, Doggett MA (1992) *Measures of Need and Outcome for Primary Health Care*. Oxford University Press, Oxford.

Computer compendiums

Tamburini M. Quality of Life Assessment in Medicine: Bibliographic Reference. This CD is updated regularly and is available from Glamm Interactive Srl, Viale Corsica 7, 20133 Milan, Italy (e-mail qlam@glamm.com).
Staquet M. Quality of Life Updated Bibliography. This 3.5 inch disk is updated regularly and is available from M Staquet, Faculty of Medicine (DCS), CP623, Route de Lennik 88808, B-1070, Brussels, Belgium.

Also, a video series on health status measurement is available from the Medical Outcomes Trust, 8 Park Plaza, Suite 503, Boston, Massachussetts, MA 02116, USA.

The journals *Quality of Life Research* and *Medical Care* publish a considerable amount on health status measurement, questionnaire design and application.

Glossary

Alpha reliability statistic A statistic used to determine the internal reliability of scales (*see* Reliability).

Ceiling and floor effects Refer to the response range and the method of scoring an instrument. Thus, an instrument applied to a random sample of the population which is not sensitive to lower levels of ill health and that is scored from 0 (good health) to 100 (poor health) would be said to manifest a floor effect, as most respondents would score 0. On the other hand if the instrument was scored from 0 (poor health) to 100 (good health) this would be referred to as a ceiling effect, as most respondents would score 100. Such floor and ceiling effects are more likely to be found in instruments with small numbers of items.

Clinical trial An experiment to assess the efficacy of a treatment.

Construct A phenomenon that exists theoretically but that cannot be measured directly and is defined or operationalized in terms of other observed indicators. Thus, it is not possible to measure depression in the same way as height, so indirect measures (questionnaires of self-report or clinical assessment of behaviour) have to be used.

Construct validity Where hypotheses are generated and a questionnaire tested to determine if it actually reflects these prior hypotheses. For example, the construct validity of the SF-36 has been checked to ensure that certain groups (e.g. older, lower social classes, those with illnesses) gain lower scores (i.e. indicating worse health) than other groups (e.g. younger, higher social classes, those without illnesses).

Content validity The extent to which items on a questionnaire tap all the relevant aspects of the attribute they are intending to measure.

Convergent and discriminant validity A measure should both converge with other indicators of the same concept and be able to discriminate unrelated indicators.

Cost-utility analysis A form of economic cost-effectiveness analysis where the effects of health care interventions are assessed according to the quality-adjusted life-years gained or lost (*see* Chapter 5, *see also* QALYs).

Criterion validity The extent to which a measure correlates with a pre-existing one, preferably a 'gold standard'. There are two types: (i) concurrent validity, where a new measure is administered at the same time as a pre-existing one, and the two are correlated, and (ii) predictive validity.

Cronbach's alpha *see* Alpha reliability statistic

Dimensions of health Theoretically or empirically distinct aspects of health, for example physical and mental health. Dimensions are also frequently referred to as 'domains'.

Disease-specific measures Questionnaires designed for use with a particular patient group, e.g. the Parkinson's Disease Questionnaire was designed exclusively for use with patients with Parkinson's disease (*see also* Generic measure).

Domain *see* Dimensions of health.

Effect size A statistic for determining the difference between scores gained at two different times. This statistic has been recommended as a method of evaluating the sensitivity of health measurement instruments to important clinical change, calculated by dividing the mean change in score by the baseline standard deviation (*see* Chapter 3; *see also* Standardized response mean, Index of responsiveness).

Face validity The need for a questionnaire to apparently tap, simply by item content, an underlying dimension. Questions should be unambiguous and easily understood and should reflect issues appropriate to the dimension.

Factor analysis A group of statistical techniques whose purpose is to reduce a large number of variables to a smaller number of latent variables, i.e. variables that cannot be measured directly. Thus a number of questions may be seen as measuring the single theoretical concept of 'anxiety'.

Floor effect *see* Ceiling and floor effects.

Generic measure A measure designed for use with any illness groups or population samples, as opposed to those intended for specific illness groups.

Guttman scaling A scale containing items, which are summed, that all tap aspects of the same phenomena. Each item contains sets of statements which are hierarchically ranked. Affirmation of a statement means that all statements below it are also affirmed and all those above it are not. Thus by affirming item number 3 in the following example then 1 and 2 must also be true, whilst 4 is not: 4. I can walk very long distances beyond a mile; 3. I can walk a mile; 2. I can walk half a mile; 1. I can walk very short distances.

Health There are numerous definitions of health, but perhaps the most widely quoted is that of the World Health Organization which claims that health is a state of complete physical, mental, and social well-being and not merely the absence of disease or infirmity.

Health index Where all the items of an instrument are summed producing one overall score, for example the EuroQol (*see* Chapter 5).

Health outcomes The end results of medical interventions and processes. These can be assessed in terms of mortality, morbidity, physiological measures and, increasingly, more subjective patient-based assessments of health.

Health profile A questionnaire covering various dimensions of health, as opposed to a health index which sums all measured aspects of health into a single figure.

Health-related quality of life This refers to an individual's level of health-related well-being. Measurement of health-related quality of life addresses the various dimensions of health (*see* Dimensions of health).

Health status A level of health in terms of physical, social and mental well-being.

Index of responsiveness A statistic for determining the difference between scores gained at two different times (*see* Chapter 3; *see also* Effect size, Standardized response mean).

Instrument In health status measurement this refers to the tool with which health status or quality of life is measured, usually in the form of a questionnaire.

Internal consistency *see* Chapter 3, Internal consistency reliability.

Internal consistency reliability Assessment of internal consistency reliability involves examining the extent to which a number of items addressing the same concept actually are doing so. There are a number of ways of calculating the correlation between items: for example, split-half reliability, whereby the measure is randomly split into two groups and reliability is assessed by the correlation between the two half tests, and Cronbach's alpha, a statistical test of internal consistency based on the mean correlation between items (*see* Chapter 3).

Inter-rater reliability Addresses the consistency of a measure when administered by different interviewers. This is tested by interviewing the same people with the same measures but using different interviewers with only a short period of time between. Kappa coefficient of agreement is the statistical tool used to assess whether differences were due to agreement or chance (*see* Chapter 3).

Interval scales It is assumed that data on an interval scale are ordered and the distances between values on one part of the scale are equal in distance to the distances between values on another part of the scale. Temperature is measured on such a scale. However, interval scales lack an absolute baseline anchorpoint. For example, a thermometer is an interval scale but it is not possible to assume that 60°F is twice as hot as 30°F, as 0°F is not as cold as it can get (*see* Chapter 3).

Item   An individual question which may stand alone or form part of a battery of questions in a dimension.

Item content   Refers to the actual wording of the individual questions. Such content must at least satisfy requirements of face validity (*see* Validity).

Latent variable   A variable that cannot be measured directly, but is measured indirectly (*see also* Construct, Factor analysis).

Likert scale   A response scale in which respondents select from a range of options which are placed on a continuum, such as Never, Rarely, Sometimes, Often, Very Often. A number of related questions tapping the aspects of the same phenomenon will, ideally, have the same response categories and can be summed.

Longitudinal study   Where individuals in a study are followed over time.

Minimally important difference   The minimally important difference (MID) is that difference in a health status measure score that corresponds to the smallest change that patients consider important (*see* Chapter 3).

Multidimensional measures   Instruments which consider health in more than one dimension/domain – for example, mobility, pain, mental health.

Nominal scales   These scales distinguish classes of objects. For example, the classification of sex into 1 = male and 2 = female is a nominal scale. A more complex nominal scale is the International Classification of Diseases, where numerical values classify all diagnoses and presenting problems. There is no hierarchy implied by the values ascribed, so in the example of sex it would be equally valid to code 1 = female and 2 = male (*see* Chapter 3)

Non-parametric methods   Statistical analyses which assume that data do not follow the normal distribution.

Normal distribution   Data that produce a 'bell curve' with the mean, mode and median all having the same value.

Normative data   Data which are representative of a population.

Ordinal scales   Classes or objects are ordered on a continuum (for example, from Best to Worst). No indication is given as to the distance between values, although a hierarchy is assumed to exist. Thus when classifying an illness into 1 = mild, 2 = moderate and 3 = severe, it cannot be assumed that the difference between mild and moderate is similar to the size of the difference between moderate and severe (*see* Chapter 3).

Parametric methods   Statistical analyses in which the data are assumed to be normally distributed.

Precision   The ability of an instrument to differentiate between illness groups or states of health.

Predictive validity   The ability of an instrument to predict some other measure of outcome.

Psychometrics   Science of measuring mental and subjective phenomena.

Quality-adjusted life-year (QALY)   A generic measure of health benefit which attempts to represent the relative value attached by society to different improvements in health, enabling systematic comparison between a variety of health care interventions. Comparisons between treatment programmes are expressed in QALYs. With a measure of both the life-years gained from a particular intervention and the quality of life in each of those years it is possible to calculate the number of QALYs obtained. Thus, an index of quality of life multiplied by the number of years in that health state equals the number of QALYs (*see* Chapter 5).

Random sample   Where each individual in the given population has an equal chance of selection into the sample.

Ratio scales   A ratio scale is an interval scale with an absolute 0 point, so that ratios between values can be meaningfully defined; thus 10 km is twice as long as 5 km. Time, weight and height are all examples of ratio scales (*see* Chapter 3).

Regression   A group of statistical techniques whose purpose is to predict the value of some variable or variables when others are known.

Reliability   A reliable measure is one which produces consistent results from the same subjects at different times when no evidence of change exists (*see* Chapter 3; *see also* Test-retest reliability, Internal consistency reliability, Inter-rater reliability).

Response range   The set of answers available to respondents for each item.

Responsiveness   The extent to which an instrument can detect change in health status over time (*see* Chapter 3; *see also* Ceiling and floor effects, Effect size, Standardized response mean, Index of responsiveness).

Scales   A graded system of categories. More frequently in psychology and health status measurement, the term refers more specifically to a series of self-report questions which can in some way be summed (*see* Chapter 3; *see also* Nominal scales, Ordinal scales, Interval scales, Ratio scales).

Sensitivity to change   An instrument's ability to detect change over time, sometimes referred to as 'responsiveness' (*see* Chapter 3).

Standardized response mean   A statistic for determining the difference between scores gained at two different times. It is calculated by dividing the mean change on a scale by the mean change in the standard deviation. Such a method is recommended when comparing the sensitivity to change of various health status measures (*see* Chapter 3; *see also* Effect size).

Subjective well-being   The patient's assessment of their own health status as opposed to professionally or clinically defined indicators.

Systematic review   A review in which the methods for selecting and including or excluding publications are explicitly stated.

Test-retest reliability   This involves the administration of an instrument on two separate occasions to the same population. The correlation between scores provides an estimate of the measure's reliability. The two occasions need to be far enough apart so that previous responses cannot be remembered but close enough in time so that change in the true score is minimal (*see* Chapter 3).

Thurstone's method of paired comparisons   A technique for gaining relative values for items on a questionnaire. Each item is judged in relation to every other item and simply assessed in terms of which of the two has more of the given property under investigation. From this procedure, weights are derived that are applied to the items. Consequently respondents tick either 'Yes' or 'No' to statements which are weighted. Thus, on the Nottingham Health Profile the item 'I cannot walk at all' gains greater value than 'I have difficulty walking about outside'.

Utility   The preference for or desirability of a particular outcome in terms of health status.

Validity   The extent to which an instrument measures the desired underlying concept (*see* Chapter 3; *see also* Face validity, Content validity, Criterion validity).

Visual analogue scale   Typically a 10 cm line on which the respondent indicates the intensity of his or her response. Phrases are printed at the ends of the line (e.g. 'No pain' and 'Extreme pain') to indicate the scope of the scale.

Weighting   Items which are given values indicating their relative importance to other items on a scale are said to be weighted. For example, on the NHP, the item 'I cannot walk at all' is given a greater value than 'I need help to walk about outside'. There is a considerable body of evidence that in many instances such weighting schemes make only marginal differences to scoring simply by addition of raw scores.

Index